SOMEWHERE IN BETWEEN

SEAN C. PIRKLE, MD

First Edition: July 2025

ISBN: 979-8-9989892-0-9 (paperback)

ISBN: 979-8-9989892-2-3 (ebook)

Library of Congress Control Number: 2025910449

Cover Design by Zuchal Rosyidin (Kamaji Studio)

Published by PirkleMD, LLC

Seattle, WA 98122

 Formatted with Vellum

For Sarah.

CONTENTS

PROLOGUE

It makes you wonder. All the brilliant things we might have done with our lives if only we suspected we knew how.

—Ann Patchett, *Bel Canto*

My heart skipped a beat when I first learned that I was delivering the commencement address at my high school graduation. I remember thinking how odd it was for an eighteen-year-old to offer kids his own age, or anyone, advice on how to live their lives. I spent the final few months of my senior year racking my brain for any nuggets of insight to leave behind.

I found that the problem with reflection was that, in so many facets of life, the journey never seemed complete. Everything I had experienced up to that point was intertwined in this giant, three-dimensional web. An action at one point in space did not just radiate from the center like ripples on the surface of a pond, but it diffused into and out of the plane at an infinite number of angles, altering the way the past was perceived and how the future would unfold, such that the impact of a singular event looked entirely different from each vantage point. And at that juncture in my high school career, I still had no idea what to make of the past four years. High school was a continuation of grade school; college would be a continuation of high school. There never really was an end. Closure either did not exist or could not be pinpointed because change came and went, and I had established new equilibriums wherever I settled. Nevertheless, after a dozen rounds of writing and rewriting, I eventually committed to a message.

On the day of commencement, I stood in front of some four thousand attendees—my classmates, our families and friends— and attempted to articulate our shared high school experience. Though I struggled to pinpoint an area of expertise in my speech, I found solace in the fact that I did not have to impart some profound thesis. I could simply talk about what I had observed over the past four years: how what we labeled meaningful as high school graduates were not the test scores that we'd achieved nor the awards we'd earned. Instead, this period of our lives would come to be defined by a collection of memories and what they meant to us: early morning practices, spirit weeks, senior pranks, that first beer. The girls we'd kissed and the ones we hadn't. Missed opportunities and missed curfews. We had established relationships capable of transcending time and space, and that was worth holding onto.

Watching a recording of that speech years later, I see a younger version of myself wearing an oversized maroon gown decorated with tassels and stoles. I nervously sway behind a podium half my size as the camera shifts focus between my face and the beach balls bouncing in the foreground. I hear a shaky voice describing scenes from my youth, attempting to avoid clichés, and when I dare to deliver my call to action, I can hear myself clearly:

> *I could say that the best is yet to come, and you would believe me. But the reality of this moment is that I don't know any better than you what the future holds.*

At that time, I had never gone to college, worked for a living, married, or started a family. I had no firsthand experience with any of those life events which people more mature than I had claimed fulfilled them. But the point I sought to impart was that what I knew then, standing in front of what felt like the world, was that there was an abundance of potential energy that came with graduation, and what we did with it was entirely up to us. In that moment, our futures seemed like a slab of marble: dark, rough, imposing, yet at the same time, completely undefined. With each decision, we had the power to chisel away and create something beautiful, to make mistakes and fix them, to learn through trial and error how to work the stone until we shaped it into our vision. The decisions we made over the next four or fourteen or forty years would define our legacies, so why would we not attempt to find our own versions of greatness? The possibilities were endless.

As I set off, trying to follow my own advice, I spent a few weeks before the start of college living with my uncle and his family, who had devoted the past few years of their lives to mission work at a community hospital and an elementary school in Balfate, Honduras. The goal was to immerse myself in the Spanish language prior to embarking on a Spanish major. I have fond memories from that summer of playing soccer with the local children, jogging home with open sores on the soles of my feet after running around barefoot all day.

One sunny afternoon, however, I found myself staring at the body of a child on a dusty bed. To this day, I cannot recall what caused his condition, but I do remember his name. I remember the sweat-stained grimace on his face, the way he contorted his body to silence the pain from his swollen limbs. The heat, the dirt, and the smell of garbage. I remember realizing that, during all the commotion of those tending to fresh wounds, a team of physicians had formed a small circle around this child, and on the outside of this circle, from the corner of the room, I stood with hands buried deep within my pockets. From there for the next hour, a rollercoaster of emotions hit me in succession: disappointment, solemnity, emptiness. But more than anything, I felt raw. Instead of springing into action for another in his time of need, I remained a passive figure, petrified by ignorance. Frozen in that corner, I absorbed this curious combination of frustration and hope and realized that I had found my purpose. Not long afterward, I enrolled in general chemistry, signed up for the Medical College Admissions Test (MCAT), and applied to medical school. My newfound passion was medicine: conducting my own research, teaching others, and above all else, healing the sick and injured.

It seems contradictory, but even after gaining acceptance to and graduating from medical school, I still often entertain this thought that a certain essence of potential has slipped from my grasp. At one time or another, we all find ourselves making choices that set our lives on completely altered trajectories. Like a steel ball rolling down Waddington's epigenetic landscape, we must evolve to pass through thresholds beyond which there is no reversal. The problem is that there is no way to consider all the possible effects of making one decision over another until it is far too late. Or at least until we perceive it is too late. The road not taken is lurking, it is haunting, it is ever present. What if I never dropped that Spanish major? What if I applied for a different summer internship? What if I weren't so impatient and took that gap year or two or three or ten? One day, an aunt at a family reunion asked me what I wanted to study in college, and I responded "premed," and there it was. The first step. Each step pulled the next along and with increasing ground traversed came increasing difficulty turning around and starting anew. It had inertia.

There's this self-fulfilling prophecy, this part of me that seeks to silence the cognitive dissonance and find a calling and vehemently justify it until I have satisfied my own worries. It's safe. I find comfort in the security that accompanies the guise of direction. Next thing I know, I am in a hospital, looking at a man with a history of high blood pressure and type 2 diabetes mellitus. In a basic science lab pipetting Dulbecco's Modified Eagle Medium (DMEM) onto self-replicating embryonic stem cells. In the waiting room of a free clinic, calling the next patient's name for their appointment. It's a strange realization to make a decision without fully understanding its gravity or permanence, to make a choice that is now synonymous with who I am, even when it is what I want.

Medicine is a defined path for at least ten years: medical school for four years, internship for one, finishing residency for another three to six, maybe a chief year or a fellowship if I end up subspecializing. Because of this, it is easy to feel as if some of the freedom I had back when I was graduating high school has vaporized; the marble slab has begun to take form. I can see hunks of stone at my ankles and the rough outline of a figure before me. Instead of forging a path on my own, it has been hacked out in a series of applications and test dates. While the pursuit of medicine requires the sacrifice of so much possibility, the forfeiture of the relentless hypotheticals we luxuriate in when we're young—that consulting internship or teaching English overseas—being a physician presents an entirely new set of possibilities which I could have never fully understood when I first started on this journey.

When I was an undergraduate at Vanderbilt University in Nashville, Tennessee, I volunteered at a medical student-run free clinic called the Shade Tree during my junior and senior years. On Saturdays, I helped the front desk by organizing patient charts and shuttling patients from one room to another. A couple of months prior to my college graduation, the supervising physician for the day held a "chalk talk" to educate the medical students, who were on their clinical rotations, as well as some of the other volunteers who, like I, had stuck around after the clinic had closed for the day. Once the team of fifteen had circled the whiteboard, the physician paused to scan the room before locking eyes with me and asking, "Sean, what do you want to learn about today?"

I panicked for a split second, furiously scanning everything I knew about medicine and the human body. After a brief silence, I looked back and said the only thing I could think of: "I don't even know what I don't know."

————

I started recording the details that would later become this book because, like that young commencement speaker or that premed volunteer, I had no idea what I was doing. My parents aren't in medicine. My dad is a commercial banker for a corporate bank that provides loans to medium-to-large-sized businesses investing in international growth. My mom is a retired contracts manager for a defense company that distributes large antennas capable of supporting Wi-Fi in remote parts of the world. She used to tell me that a contracts manger was a glorified customer service representative for executives in the Middle East. She didn't like that job, but the pay was reasonable and, more importantly, the hours were flexible enough to allow her to drive her two kids to practices and back and put microwavable dinners on the table.

In fact, I come from a long line of people who excelled in fields very different than medicine. My dad's dad trained in theology, and he had taken a position for many years as the dean of students at a private Christian college in Mobile, Alabama. His father before him owned a small farm in South Georgia which harvested an assortment of crops, including watermelons, cantaloupe, peanuts, and cotton.

My mom's dad provided for his wife and two children with an information technology salary. I was told he "kept the computers running" in a city-state now known as Singapore, which had only recently freed itself from British colonialism at the time he was entering the workforce. My grandmothers had supported their families in more traditional roles as homemakers and schoolteachers.

I was one of a few in my extended family to attend post-graduate school focused on the sciences, and the first in my nuclear family to attend medical school. By way of this background, the idea behind this memoir was to provide a tell-all documentation of what it was like to go to medical school, because I wanted other people in my shoes to not be burdened with this uncertainty about what lay ahead. I think, in many ways, this book is for them, and for the younger version of myself who was confused and intimidated by the logistical hurdles and sacrifice required to become qualified to care for another human life.

This book was written over the course of four years in the early morning hours, after midterm exams, and on flights home for Thanksgiving and Christmas. I think it succeeds at painting in larger brushstrokes what the day-to-day of medical training can be like, with an understanding that medicine remains a rapidly evolving field, and that the minutiae will change over time. What I did not expect from this period in my life was how the process of learning how to doctor coincided with attempting to learn how to be an adult. During the most formative period in my life, I experienced adversity I could have never predicted. I was labelled with new medical diagnoses, and I went through breakups and found new love. I met individuals who changed the way I observe and now experience the world. I had my future dangled in front of me by a computer algorithm and was forced to figure out what I actually wanted from this life. This book has grown into so much more than just a snapshot of modern-day medical training, and I invite readers from all backgrounds to experience with me this journey which includes becoming a doctor, a patient, a partner, and a citizen of this Earth.

MS1

1

WHITE COAT

Let us suppose the mind to be, as we say, white paper, void of all characters.

—John Locke

I COULD HEAR the cicadas buzzing, their song braided with the hum of the power lines above. The Chicago summer was hot and humid, and I had to concentrate to not work up a sweat on the walk down South Greenwood Avenue. Accompanying me were my sister and parents, who had traveled from the mountains of North Georgia to celebrate with me, as well as my new roommates and their families, whom I had met the week prior. Ryan had driven in from the neighboring Midwestern city of Cincinnati, Ohio. Jason flew in from Portland, Oregon, and Russell had grown up just a short train ride north of New York, New York. The four of us had spent the previous week and a half shuttling Honda Accord-sized loads of kitchen appliances, coffee tables, and barstools from Ikea and back, slowly furnishing the four-bedroom walk-up apartment that would be our home for the next four years.

When we arrived at the main quad, we took in the ivy clinging to the façade of Ida Noyes Hall, and with a deep breath, welcomed the cool air as we entered the atrium to join the remaining eighty-four members of our medical school class. At orientation that week, I learned that my classmates had come from all corners of the United States and abroad. Many, like I, had gone straight through college to medical school, while others had tried out different careers in accounting, consulting, and investment banking prior to deciding on medicine. Among us, there were Fulbright Scholars, former college student body presidents, semi-professional athletes, Peace Corps volunteers, Teach for America instructors, and PhDs. I would later become lifelong friends with many of these individuals, my forever advisors for questions on topics ranging from high blood pressure medications to pediatric milestones, and others would stand beside me as groomsmen and bridesmaids on my wedding day.

We all seemed to share the same nervous energy, and our small talk about the architectural boat cruise we had taken the day before was soon interrupted with directions on when and how to walk down the aisle, single file. We beamed at our families as we passed them, and they returned our enthusiasm with frenetic waving. When we were seated, several speakers stood onstage and delivered a lifetime of advice nobody would remember, and afterward, they called us up to join them and receive our first piece of professional paraphernalia: the white coat.

The White Coat Ceremony is perhaps the most recognizable

tradition from the first year of medical school, and you may be surprised to learn that the tradition is one of medicine's youngest. What initially started in 1989 in the very hall where I received my white coat has now grown into an honored ritual at over one hundred schools across the US, including many dental, pharmacy, and physician assistant schools. The ceremony lets new health professions students celebrate kicking off a career dedicated to compassion, competence, and the relentless pursuit of scientific knowledge. While its practical significance may have diminished since the days of early medicine, the power of the white coat continues to inspire and reassure patients, and if nothing else, creep its way into the Instagram feeds of all intrepid medical students.

After receiving our coats, we were directed back to our seats to recite a modified version of the oath our physician ancestors had taken since 400 BCE, words we were pledging to live by for the remainder of our years in practice:

> *I will be just and generous to those who have taught*
> *me this art, holding them in the highest esteem,*
> *and will give guidance and instruction freely to all*
> *who wish to follow in this path.*
> *I will strive to extend its domain, while remembering*
> *that medicine is more than science, and that*
> *warmth, sympathy, and understanding may heal*
> *as well as the surgeon's knife or the chemist's drug.*
> *I will practice my art solely for the benefit of my*
> *patients, knowing that at times I must put their*
> *interests before my own. May I never see in my*
> *patient anything but a fellow human in pain. My*
> *goal will be to help, or at least do no harm.*

*I will remain free of all intentional injustice, prac-
ticing with integrity and honor, and will not
exploit my privileged role in the lives of my
patients. What is revealed to me in confidence, I
will keep inviolably secret. I will use my skills to
serve all in need, with openness of spirit and
without bias.*

*In the presence of my teachers, my family, and my
friends, I make this pledge freely and upon my
honor. I am ready for my vocation now and I turn
unto my calling.*

I hung onto every syllable of the Hippocratic Oath as it rolled out of my mouth, realizing that I could finally see myself as a doctor. It was one of those moments so filled with wonder that I wish it would have crystalized, so that I could have plucked it out of thin air to reference when the details faded.

I remained floating in a glass bubble of appreciation and exhilaration until an intrusive thought shattered it. While the White Coat Ceremony was the chance to finally envision what I had been working toward for years, a moment of brief accomplishment before the start of something entirely novel, I was reminded many times over that day that this was more than a celebration of what we had achieved. With the donning of the white coat came the responsibility of what it embodied, and sitting on the hardwood benches where it all began, I could not help but start to feel an earnest agreement with what our keynote speaker described as a "foreboding concern for what comes next."

What came over the next few months—as coursework in anatomy, physiology, clinical skills, and methods of inquiry revved up—was a realization that patients' lives would, in the not-so-distant future, be in my hands. This meant that the information I was cramming into my brain was no longer for my own sake but for the betterment of future patient lives. I found this to be particularly horrifying because I was acutely aware that, when it came down to where I was in my life, despite what I had tried to feign to my non-premed friends throughout my college years, at the start of medical school, I knew absolutely nothing about medicine. This feeling, unfortunately, had been validated on numerous occasions by the dozens of rejections I had endured during the medical school application cycle and, more recently, by being waitlisted by the school in which I eventually, albeit just recently, enrolled.

———

The process of gaining acceptance to medical school is not for the faint of heart. It requires a strong grade point average in undergraduate courses, studying for months on end and subsequently excelling at the MCAT, and participation in a host of extracurricular activities, such as research, sports, or club leadership roles. After submitting application materials—including a personal statement, college transcripts, test scores, and letters of recommendation—most schools will send back a secondary application sometime thereafter with a few essay prompts specific to their institution. Most attempt to get at the culture of what they are trying to promote: "What does diversity mean to you?" "Tell me about a time you were faced with adversity." "Share an experience when you failed and how you handled it."

If the tangibles of the application and the intangibles of the secondary responses are up to their standards, schools may offer a qualified prospective student an in-person interview.

One of my first interviews for medical school was at the University of Pittsburgh. In the days leading up to the interview, I had traded emails with a first-year medical student (MSI) who had volunteered to host me. Hosting programs such as this were standard practice shared by most medical schools, a way to help prospects cut costs on an otherwise expensive interview trail consisting of last-minute plane rides and Ubers to and from campus. At the time, it was so bizarre to me, traveling to a new city by myself and being a guest in a stranger's home, but there I was, twenty-one and anxious, doing the thing.

I arrived at my host's apartment late on a Sunday. From the living room, on the couch which doubled as my bed for the night, we made conversation about the unique qualities of Pitt's medical education, the school's culture, and the way the movie *Perks of Being a Wallflower* so accurately portrayed the tunnel heading into the City of Bridges—how when my car carved its way through the mountain before hitting the Monongahela River on the other side, it was neither day nor night and, for those fifteen seconds, before our ejection from the halogen light into the most breathtaking view of the skyline, life felt infinite.

I met his roommate later that evening, before we all went our separate ways, me to my couch, my host to his bed upstairs, and the roommate to his room on the lower level. I was told if I needed to use the toilet, I could use the bathroom downstairs, which was accessible by exiting through the back door on the main level out onto the deck, walking down the wooden stairs, and re-entering the home through the basement. Alternatively, one could walk down the stairs in the living room, directly into the second bedroom, and out the door on the adjacent wall. This was the route the roommate took to beat me to brushing my teeth.

I slept about as well as I could have hoped, and as I did before all my interviews, I awoke at dawn, ready to get the day started. I grabbed my toiletry kit and went to shower, walking out the back door and entering the basement as instructed. When finished, I wrapped myself in a towel I had brought from home and made my way inside, the whole time aware of the water droplets I had missed on my exposed back, each individual bead serving as a reminder of the crisp autumn morning air.

As I approached the back door of the living room, I could see my suit still hanging where I left it, but when I went to turn the knob, it did not budge. I squeezed tighter and turned with more fervor, but the results were no different. Confused, I peered in through the kitchen window, and noticed that the dead bolt had inexplicably turned in the ten minutes I was downstairs. At this hour, nobody else in the house was awake, but still I tried knocking, to no avail. I could no longer deny it: I was trapped outside a random person's home, wet, freezing, and wearing nothing but a towel. One million thoughts went through my head, but a decision had to be made. The solution in my mind was clear. I walked back downstairs and entered through the basement. I looked at the only other closed door down there and took a deep breath before entering.

I knew the door would creak open; the hinges had rusted over in this industrial, late 1970s townhome. To open quickly like a Band-Aid or slowly and smoothly was the most important choice of my life in that moment, and after a beat of contemplation, I elected to be deliberate and gradual. I cringed, this time as the door yielded to my grasp, the bottom brushing the carpet as it eased open. When I peeked my head through the crack, I saw my host's roommate fast asleep under the covers. I tiptoed around his bed, the fifteen feet to the other door feeling like a mile, and in a blink, I made it to the other side. I quickly slunk out the other door and scampered up the stairs to the main room before changing into my suit. At breakfast, I greeted my host and his roommate and did not say a word about the previous hour's expedition. I interviewed a few hours later and was rejected from the medical school a few months after that.

I interviewed at Cornell on my birthday. When I was first invited, I was thrilled. While the college was situated in Upstate New York, the medical campus was located on the Upper East Side of Manhattan. During my sophomore year of college, I had spent a summer living in Kips Bay, on twenty-third and third, participating in a research fellowship at New York University. From this experience, I knew I was the kind of person who could appreciate the good (halal stands are open at 2:00 a.m.!) and the bad (getting hit by trash water raining from the window units of high-rise apartments) of the Big Apple, and I was excited to have the opportunity to potentially start my medical education there. It did not take living in New York City, though, to know that the cost of living was bordering on inhospitable. Despite this, and to my surprise, Cornell did not have a student hosting program like Pitt's. As a result, I was left to my own devices to find housing the night before my interview. Not wanting to spend an exorbitant amount of money on a hotel, I booked a hostel across Central Park on the Upper West Side. When I arrived, I knew I'd made a horrible mistake.

The room I had reserved was shared with twelve others. The cast of characters outwardly appeared to have nothing in common, but regardless of from whence they came, the stench was nevertheless the same. I slept with a determination to thwart thieves, the strap of my weekender bag looped around my leg and my cellphone clutched to my chest. It vibrated me awake around 5:00 a.m. and I was dressed and ready to go well before my interviews. After breakfast, I called a cab to shuttle me across the park to the hospital campus. What I failed to account for was that the United Nations was in town for an assembly, and as a result, multiple streets were closed to through traffic. I sat in a standstill for over an hour, frantically updating the admissions coordinator as to my whereabouts, as my interview time came and went. I eventually showed up thirty minutes after my first scheduled interview and was rejected from the medical school a few months after that.

The Mayo Clinic is essentially the pinnacle of modern medicine. It has a longstanding tradition of excellence, and every year, patients fly from all over the world to receive treatment there. Because of this reputation, I was not surprised when I was sweating twenty minutes into my first thirty-minute interview. Despite interviewing toward the end of my cycle, this was by far the most difficult one I had attended.

"You seem to have a really strong connection with your sister. What is your favorite quality of hers?"

Months prior to this interview, I had applied to over twenty programs. Given the sheer volume of secondary essays I had written for all of these schools, I did not remember what information I had shared with each one, but I was fairly certain that I had not said anything about my older sister anywhere on my application. Since they were asking, though, I knew I must have, or in any case, they were aware that this relationship existed, and I was left telling them how I loved that she was always able to find a way to connect with other people. It was true, I did admire that about her.

"I think we all have different experiences with mortality, and I enjoyed reading about your perspective. Can you tell me, Sean, when you die, what do you hope is on your epitaph?"

I punted this one as well and made up something about how I hoped to be remembered as a genuinely good person whose influence on the world was net positive. Yikes.

And the kicker: "It was brave of you to talk about your struggle with bulimia on this application. Can you speak a little more about this journey?"

I balked, "I'm not bulimic...?"

At this, the interviewer looked down and laughed. "Oh my goodness, my apologies! I've been looking at the wrong application the whole time."

I finished the remaining ten minutes of my interview with questions about topics that I had included on my application, and I was rejected from the medical school a few months after that.

———

Despite the many schools that, after much consideration, regretted to inform me they could not offer me a place in their class, I was ultimately accepted by the University of Chicago Pritzker School of Medicine. After a long application cycle spent waiting, then packing, then moving, I sat in Ida Noyes with a heart full of gratitude and a head full of doubt, surrounded by Ivy League students to the left, former All-Americans to the right, nobody in front of me because that student had been excused from orientation to fly across the Atlantic Ocean and present research in Cambridge—incredible human beings who held accolades which I could never, in a lifetime, earn. Drowning in this environment of high achievers, pondering my self-worth, it was hard to not feel like an outsider playing dress-up in an oversized, medium starch white coat.

When I was three, my parents moved me and my sister to Forsyth County, a middle-class suburb of Atlanta, Georgia, where, less than a decade prior to our arrival, the Ku Klux Klan still haunted the streets. Here, I grew up in classrooms where every student was the same hue and where all of my teachers shared this background. As a kid looking around, being forced to grapple with the notion that I was the only person in the room who looked like me, I honestly wished I could have blended in. On standardized tests, when surveyed about race, I filled in the bubble marked "White," hoping it would be true. Every now and again, I would step onto the baseball diamond and be reminded of this falsity, fielding chants of "Jackie Chan" and "Ichiro Suzuki" as they echoed out of opposing teams' dugouts. When I graduated high school, my peers whispered that I was only admitted to Vanderbilt University because I was a minority.

I have been othered at times during my life, and because of this, the feeling was nothing foreign. Before medical school started, though, I had never really felt isolated in an academic sense. School had always come easily to me. I'd excelled since I was little. High school was a relative breeze. After bombing the first two assignments of my freshman year of college—a General Chemistry lab safety quiz (75 percent, woof) and a Calculus 1 exam (68 percent, R.I.P.)—I stopped binge drinking cheap vodka on Thursday nights and figured out how to study.

But during the first few months of medical school, I would

be frequently inundated with information I had never seen before. I'd find myself surrounded by people who seemed more intelligent, more competent—simply put, better students, better speakers, just *better* than me. It'd be so obvious to me that I had no idea what I was doing, and I'd occasionally deliberate whether I was only there to fill some kind of quota. But if that were true, then what diverse perspective did I even bring? How many others in my cohort were last-minute additions off the waitlist? Who else was profoundly worried that they'd failed the cardiopulmonary resuscitation (CPR) training post-test that we had taken at orientation? How many others were still reeling from Reviewer #2's feedback on their second ever manuscript submission to an academic journal demanding that they "do better science"?

The trek home from Ida Noyes felt much longer than the walk there. Dusk came and my parents flew back to their home tucked away at the base of the Appalachian Mountains, and I was left alone to organize the shoeboxes of mementos I had salvaged from previous lives: a baseball with signatures of the 9U team I'd coached in college, a wooden ping-pong paddle from my childhood home, a corkboard littered with ticket stubs from the University of Georgia football wins over Auburn, Florida, and Tennessee.

I picked the white coat up off my bed and placed a pin from the Shade Tree Clinic on the lapel as a reminder of how far I had come. I hung it delicately on an extra hanger and tucked it away in the corner of my closet for another day, and though I wasn't *really*, I couldn't help but feel alone. I had uprooted my life and started over in a new city where I didn't have any friends or family. I had put myself in this position where I knew I'd feel inadequate each day, and when I understood that my curriculum vitae of failures was much longer than that of my successes, it was hard to be convinced that the shorter list was more meaningful.

With the door to my bedroom closed, I could hear excited chatter coming from the common area. My peers were talking about the next day's classes and their specialty interests and making jokes about how the tallest person in the class couldn't get into his white coat because it was too small. I sat on my bed eavesdropping on these conversations and contemplated for a moment that perhaps I didn't want to define my value by my peers' accomplishments. At the end of the day, no matter what we had done in our pasts to bring us together, we had all entered the same auditorium and put on the same white coat. As I turned the knob to join my roommates in the living room, I decided that what the white coat could symbolize for me was a blank slate, a new beginning, and a chance to define the person and physician that I wanted to be.

2

BAY C, STATION 17

We are all equal in the presence of death.

—Publilius Syrus

THE FIRST THING I noticed were the mops. I could see them peeking through the small, rectangular window from the other side of the door. Unamused, I pushed ahead, walking through the entrance into the fragrant perfume of formaldehyde. The smell enveloped me like that of wet paint, only this time stickier and more suffocating, finding its way into my hair, my contacts, taking root in the pores of my skin.

We were instructed to take a moment to familiarize ourselves with the new space—it was here where we would spend a substantial portion of the next eleven weeks. As we were told, we walked around the room exploring each of the four bays, inspecting the surgical lamps overhead, tinkering with the tablets decorating the walls around us, each projecting onto a pair of high-definition, 42-inch Samsung televisions at their respective stations. The walls not covered with technology were coated in a thin film of glossy primer. Expo marker-ed atop this layer were pathways of blood, lymph, and nerves littered alongside an endless list of mnemonic devices. Sunshine bounded in through the fourth-floor windows, past the human-sized black bags, casting shadows of 3D printed skulls and femurs on the tables the bags rested on, mixing a natural yellow with the fluorescent white from overhead.

But my eyes kept drifting back to the bags. Six of them were designated for each of the four bays. Each bag was situated atop a stainless steel gurney, and a metal pail dangled carelessly underneath. Beside each table, a keyboard was connected to the monitor overhead, and next to it was a neon trash bin with "#17" plastered on the side. Toward the outer margins of the corresponding bag, a zipper ran the full six feet lengthwise before making a hard left turn, effectively looping its way across the front surface of the bag toward its final destination. Enclosed underneath this zipper's teeth was the corpse assigned to me for gross anatomy lab. A team of four students, myself included, would work throughout the academic quarter to learn much about the human body from this individual.

As much as I tried to soak in the facility in its entirety, distracting me from the novelty of the environment was my own version of Schrodinger's box. Sneaking, no, storming into my consciousness was the thought that the obscured person before me was somehow both dead and alive, and the slow and labored exposition of the body within would be the simple act confirming or denying their fate. Entombed in a sheath of black plastic, they were all who had ever had the misfortune of dying and, simultaneously, nobody at all, insofar as all the bags were identical, massive silhouettes copied and pasted one after another into neat little columns in the cadaver lab of the Biological Sciences Learning Center (BSLC). Unknown to us were their faces, their stories, or even our realization of their impermanence, and the not knowing gnawed away at my psyche until it was like a grotesque Christmas trying to guess what the present was before opening it, simply judging by the shape of the box and how it sounded when shaken. Only instead of probing with my hands, I devoured it with my eyes, studying the way the bag draped coarsely over each indention and protrusion. What was their name? Were they a man or a woman? I wonder how old they *were*.

I disliked myself for the inexplicable variety of thoughts that ran through my head, feeling as though the very act of their inception was somehow disrespectful. Despite the uneasiness, I also found myself overcome with wonder: I felt a deep appreciation for how this was the most generous action of which I had personally been the recipient. The nebulous figure in front of me, in their fading moments on Earth, had chosen to donate their flesh for the advancement of a stranger's medical education, and that stranger was me. I stood in acknowledgement of this ultimate, sacred donation, an anatomical gift worthy of a moment of silence prior to the first official day of lab known colloquially as "First Cut Day." During this minute, I thanked my cadaver for their generosity. I prayed to never treat them with disrespect, to always value their life as if it were my own, to not be desensitized to their plight, and to recognize in them my own fateful mortality. Our administrators went to great lengths to ease us into this process, claiming that everybody's first encounter with cadavers is different. Some feel remorse or anguish, while others find indifference or even humor. All these emotions, we were told, were okay because we all process mortality differently.

This was, however, not my first encounter with death. I have, like most, had members of my extended family pass away. Several years ago, my great grandfather, and the Pirkle family patriarch, passed after multiple years of steady decline. He was ninety-five when his heart stopped beating, and his caretakers were relieved more than anything to see him go. From what I understood at the time, his last days were filled with pain, emotional swings, and dementia. Slowly, as disease ran its course, he had morphed into a person we had never seen before. Death had reached a stage that it no longer frightened me. Rather, it was an emancipation of his soul from the shackles of his skin. A few days after his death, the man in the casket, whom I called Grandbeaver, was no longer crumpled up on a fifty-year-old sofa scolding a nurse. He was in his best suit, clean, and with a peaceful disposition. He was a devout man, and we were all convinced he was now in a better place, a place with no more agony, reunited with his first and second wives, resting in the very heaven he had spent a lifetime believing in. It was a beautiful day and a beautiful reception. Everyone in the church was quiet. We followed the coffin out into the graveyard, and I watched as he was carefully lowered into the ground. Nobody knew exactly what to say.

The same summer that my great grandfather passed away, I completed a research program at New York University. As part of the program, we had an opportunity to spend a day down the block from the main hospital with the Manhattan medical examiner, observing autopsies of the city's homeless and indigent people. On the bottom floor of a building on 26th street, gone were the suits, the somber atmosphere, the flowers, the tears. Some of the individuals we observed were elderly and died alone, discovered only by their neighbors due to the unrelenting stench of death. Others were my age, victims of the growing opioid epidemic or chronic depression. Because the bodies were typically discovered after physical or biological abuse, they were often in poor condition. Their bodies had been mutilated by fungus or concrete or lead projectiles, and on the morning of my visit, I felt no despondency, only dread.

After changing out of chinos and a gingham button-up into a full suit of personal protective equipment, I walked into a large, open room and saw a sight I'd flash back to in that first week of anatomy lab: the same surgical lamps as in the BSLC, the same easy to clean tile floors, the same terrified look on the faces of all the visitors. Upon entering, I learned the reason behind the looks on their faces, as I was greeted by five pea green bodies spread out on five separate tables. A friend tapped me on the shoulder to make a comment about the triage we had witnessed minutes prior, and when I turned around there was already a Y-shaped lesion spanning the entirety of the chest in front of me. A few seconds later, one of the examiners pulled out a tool I had previously only seen used to trim errant tree branches from the yard of my childhood home, only the branches in this case were not privet, and as the shears clamped down, hard and fast, the splintering was not from wood but from the cracking of human ribs, removed to expose answers only the vital organs could provide. I could not fault the medical examiners for their haste—they were, after all, a well-trained assembly line. They had figured out how to harvest samples of body parts and ladle fluids into bags with impressive efficiency. I considered for a moment that what could be interpreted as apparent detachment stemmed more likely from the seemingly interminable number of bodies needing to be processed, and the unending list of questions which only their service could answer.

Still, years later on First Cut Day, when we finally unzipped the bag, I gasped. First from the sight, then from the penetrating whiff of embalming fluid. To preserve each cadaver, the bodies had been prepped in a cocktail of noxious chemicals (formalde-hyde, methanol, etc.). Whom I saw resembled a woman in form. She looked to be around five feet five inches tall. She was over-weight, and her excess abdominal tissue would have spilled over the waistband of jeans had she been wearing clothes. She had fuchsia toenails and a bandage on the index finger of her right hand that looked so *real*. Her face was wrinkled in a way that told me it belonged to a person who had lived a life worth living, but something was notably awry. It wasn't just that she was not alive, it was as if she had the life sucked out of her—hair, feces, and blood, even the pigment in her skin—to the point that I could not say with confidence whether my donor was Black, White, Asian, or Hispanic. She seemed to share the same anony-mous quality of the bag she arrived in, de-identified, but only halfway, simultaneously something I was and something I was not.

As I gingerly peeled back the bag in its entirety, I could see that her body was degraded in some places, her skin blistered into brownish-black bubbles in others. She had ropes tied around her arms, which I imagined was for transporting her rigidly flaccid body. A tag with a barcode was strapped to her wrist. Her limbs were cold, stiff, wet, and unusually pliable, with skin the consistency of wet clay.

It was no lie that each of us handled the situation uniquely. I stood staring at her body for a while, trying to emblazon this feeling in my mind. Others tackled the task at hand.

We first soaked towels in chlorine water and gently placed them around her hands, feet, and face to prevent her body from prematurely decaying. Following the instruction of our peer educators, my three teammates and I then struggled to roll 150 pounds of dead weight onto her side. We took a brief pause to catch our breaths before manipulating the forces of momentum and gravity to allow her to tumble over and settle, facedown. We then zipped up the bag and went back to our histology lecture four doors down the hallway. The job, prepping her for the next day's dissection of the back, was done.

After the first day, I noticed a dramatic shift. Each new day was a new dissection, but individually, they were simply another day in the lab. This was my new normal, and while it was anything but normal in isolation, when we did this every day for three to six hours a day, it certainly felt normal. *This was my life now*. For better or worse, we adapted astoundingly. We figured out a way to make it work. In our team of four, two dissectors would do most of the cutting. Another person would read the instructions for the day, and the fourth would either walk around the lab looking at structures in the other bays or quiz the other three group members on previous lectures, medical imaging, or osteology. We figured out who liked to do which role and settled into these positions. We learned how to be a well-functioning team not unlike the medical examiners, extracting information from the vessels before us. The atmosphere took on an appreciably lighter tone. Somebody made a penis joke as we studied the corpus cavernosum. Another referred to the perineal body as the "gooch" as we stared inches away from and into the abyss of ischioanal fossa. One day, my classmates took group pictures in their scrubs on the iPads in front of a background of Expo markings, and music eventually started playing from the computers:

> *I been on the low, I been taking my time*
> *I feel like I'm out of my mind*
> *It feel like my life ain't mine (Who can relate? Woo)*

As each new day unfolded, we recognized the deviation in our behaviors and how this was anything but funeral etiquette. But with each passing day, we told ourselves that this was also not a funeral. If it were, we would be monsters, but somehow in this room and in this particular setting, there was a way in which these actions and reverence could coexist. And we proceeded in this way for quite some time, cleaning, staring, smelling, rolling, drilling, and sawing, finding normalcy in what we were doing through it all, if only to preserve our own sanity. Within the first few weeks of medical school, we'd been forced to confront an exceedingly stark mortality and engage with it entirely, getting wrist-deep inside the tissue of another person, having her fluids splash into our hair, on our clothes, and on bad days, into our gaping mouths. If we could not normalize this, then we could not learn. If we could not learn, then we failed to gain from our cadavers the exact thing they donated their bodies for, the advancement of our medical education. So, we played music, took selfies, and made jokes about what we were doing because we didn't want to think about what we were doing any more than necessary to learn the material. It would be an exhausting and unsustainable choice. Instead, we took the path of least resistance and occupied our thoughts with lighter subjects, like weekend plans, budding relationships, or the inevitable Chicago cold that was creeping toward us with each passing day.

Our constructed truth was that the cadavers were no longer as human as they were on the first day. They did not smell nearly as bad as they once did, even though they definitely did. With each new module they lost more and more tissue, more and more organs, more and more limbs into the neon bins underneath. We had found a way to construct walls, separating what we were doing from our conception of what it was we were doing, and this transformation strengthened us. Here we were, extracting and applying information that we finally wanted to learn. This was why we were still in school, taking on debt and sacrificing weekends to textbooks. We were passionate about the material, and it refreshed us: I used a hammer and a chisel to perform a laminectomy. I dissected and reflected the muscles of the back, held two lungs in my outstretched arms. I will never forget what it's like to stick my hands into another person's chest, to reach in and wrap my fingers around the four chambers of a human heart; to feel the weight of a brain, to balance in my hands their consciousness, their sense of self and what it was that allowed souls to interact with the world; to experience love and suffering and everything in between. The complexity of the human body was awe-inspiring, and I had the privilege of discovering this in a new way each day. Even on the boring days, I found myself mindlessly defining fascial planes, cleaning up structures from the previous labs.

While we manufactured a level of comfort that I never thought would be possible, I was surprised by the way our cadavers still managed to impact us. Believe it or not, we sympathized with the pain they went through. As I made my way through the thorax, I saw the remnants of past surgeries: pacemakers and sutures. Bodies next to mine had chemotherapy delivery systems embedded beneath their skin. The further we progressed through the units, the more information we gathered. One body had an abdominal aneurism the size of a baseball, another a massive inguinal hernia protruding into his scrotum, still others had amputations from advanced diabetes. And there was so much cancer. Of the lungs, ovaries, esophagus. It was all over the room. Day by day, we came to know a little more about these people in their final moments. We established these one-dimensional relationships that could only be possible in this way, and we grew saddened by the adversity that mandated their suffering. We pondered their plight, if only for a few seconds, before shaking our heads and pushing though to find the next structure. "I cannot imagine what they were going through" was followed by, "Hey! Come look at my cadaver. He has a really interesting tumor."

I could not help but fight this constant battle between growing confidence in what I was doing and disgust with the progress I was realizing at the expense of another. I felt upset for not feeling disturbed. Guilty for enjoying the work. Uncomfortable with the ravenous hunger stimulated by a combination of inhaled formaldehyde and three straight hours of standing. And the second iteration of disgust, distress, and guilt was somehow exceeding emptiness when the question of human spirituality and eternity crept in. Navigating this dichotomy was complicated, confusing, precious even, and we had to find a balance between desensitized nonchalance and paralysis from the stark reality of what it was we were doing, which could be monstrous. I had to keep reminding myself of this fact. Nowhere else would this have been okay.

This back and forth came to a head, literally, on the first day of the penultimate module: head and neck. Until this point, our cadavers had still worn the chlorine-soaked bag which aided in preserving their face from further deterioration. It had been nearly two months of this faceless dissection of the lower limbs and pelvis, and we had grown accustomed to it—even dependent on it. Regimentation was our emotional wall; the bag was our physical wall. When it was removed, I was forced to confront the lie I had all been telling myself since the start of the course: *This is just another day. This is normal.*

Two months of gravity and many more of death had not been kind. I had since rotated to another cadaver (a new technique that my medical school employed in the curriculum to expose us to the slight variations in anatomy from human to human), so this man, while in my company for months, was quite literally a new face to me. He lay on his back, lips sealed shut, pressed flat by the unforgiving nature of the gurney. His gaze was fixed on the ceiling, brow furrowed in a brazen challenge of my next move.

I raised my scalpel, as directed in the technique guide, and aimed it where the medial border of the eye socket and the nares come together, using a vertical slit as my landing point where the skin involutes like tectonic plates between the eyes when one concentrates. As my blade slid through the layers of scalp, skin, dense connective tissue, aponeurosis, loose areolar connective tissue, down into bone, the periosteum, I expected blood to come pouring out. Congealed as it was, it refused. Somehow surprised by the lack of bleeding, I continued around the crest of his forehead, bisecting crow's feet situated atop high cheekbones, down the curve of his face through canyons of smile lines and eventually under his chin, shaving off stray whiskers as I made my trek southbound. I forced myself to steal a glimpse of the displeasure on his face, to imagine what he must be thinking, even though I knew as well as anybody that his brain was siloed off in a bucket a few feet away from his skull. I labored to continue, carefully peeling back the epidermis around his eyes, looking for the orbicularis oculi, the thin sheet of muscle responsible for the unconscious closure of our eyelids during blinking and sleep. I tugged a little too hard and pulled open his eyelid to reveal a flash of his cloudy lens looking back up into mine. For three hours, I chiseled away, and no matter how desperately I tried to speed it up, there was always more work to be done. He was always looking up with that same painstaking expression on his face. That same tortured look. Teeth clenched, biting through his tongue on both sides, eyes pleading up at me.

———

One lunch break during anatomy, I stumbled upon an *Esquire* article about the aftermath of the terrorist attacks of September 11, 2001. Titled "The Falling Man," it rehashed the day while introducing the reader to a once iconic image now buried in history.

The picture, also called "The Falling Man," had managed to capture the moment when one of the many jumpers from the Twin Towers hurtled through the air in a desperate act of survival. This man frozen in time, however, did not appear to fear death. He embraced it. He plunged toward the earth head on, arms by his side with outstretched fingers, tie flailing behind him. The portrait made it around the world overnight, eventually finding its way into *The New York Times* the following day. As Tom Junod, the article's author points out, newspapers that printed the image received countless complaints and were forced to defend themselves against accusations that they'd exploited a man's death and simultaneously robbed him and his family of privacy. Newscasts followed suit and soon began blurring out the faces of those forced out of the buildings, then not airing the images at all.

And while the jumpers' stories slowly faded out of the public consciousness due to a combination of respect, backlash, and censorship, the famous image briefly made a resurgence. Artist Eric Fischl had been commissioned in September of 2002 to make a piece for a concourse in Rockefeller Center. He chose to adapt a related image into what he called "The Tumbling Woman." Cast in bronze, the life-size sculpture was meant to portray, in his words, "something about the way we all feel" following 9/11. The sculpture only lasted a week before being taken down.

While the sharing of "The Falling Man" and the creation of "The Tumbling Woman" reflect society's desire to commemorate the victims, honor the heroes, and move forward in the face of loss, they also raise questions about the nature of remembrance and the role of disturbing images in shaping our understanding of history. Monuments representing public suffering and featuring human faces have existed for centuries, but commemorating humans in the moment of death reduces individuals to this act of terror. Here, the loss of innocent lives was captured at their most helpless, as the blameless victims of violence. I think this was why the most poignant editorials coming out of 9/11 are the ones that discuss the tiny, seemingly insignificant aspects of life that characterize lost individuals as humans. An orange toothbrush. The daily crossword. An obsession with Notre Dame football. Details that demonstrate how a person existed

with others and occupied space, how they had ideas and personalities worth remembering.

The images of those falling people may be too visceral for
many to stomach. Similarly, it may not feel right to reduce a
person's life to their moment of death because they are much
more than who they were in their waning moments. What is
hard in the anatomy lab is that we only get to know our cadavers
in death. We can explore the contents of the carpal tunnel,
marvel at how this human being had beautifully slender fingers
and wonder if they used them to play Tchaikovsky on the piano
or wield an orange toothbrush, but it will always be just that, a
curiosity.

––––––

When we pulled the bag off and exposed my cadaver's face, I
could not help but see a body and think of the life intimately
attached to it. The walls came crumbling down, and the water
came rushing in, grabbing me by the ankles and whisking me
out in the undertow. I was drowning in a sea of humanity,
reminded that there was a human face to the tragedy before me.
When lab ended, I went for a run for the first time in months. I
stepped onto the treadmill at zero, pushed the dial up to six
miles per hour, then seven, then eight until I could go no faster.
As I ran, sweat dripped down my face. It beaded on my forehead
and rolled between my eyes, downward into the crevice of my
nose, where it joined the salty tears accumulating on my cheeks.

Like so much of the public outcry following images of histor-
ical tragedies, later that night, I chose to shut out the pain. The
sun set and the doors locked, and I went home and watched
John Oliver on HBO. I went to class the next day, forgetting the

emotional troughs of the previous twenty-four hours. This time, the eyeball. The next day, the throat. Then, a full-on hemisection of the face. I lost the physical wall, but I didn't need it anymore. The emotional wall was back up and fortified tenfold, the chatter resumed. The music played softly at first, then loudly. I can still hear it:

> *Somethin' 'bout you makes me feel like a dangerous*
> *woman*
> *Somethin' 'bout, somethin' 'bout, somethin' 'bout you*

This juxtaposition is hysterical. It is both comical and senseless. A soundtrack seemingly mocking our steadfast resilience. When anatomy ended, I gathered the remnants of my cadaver and put him, piece by piece, back together into his enormous black bag. Lungs go in the chest, liver on the right, spleen on the left. The fat and fascia and skin stayed tightly sealed in their own garbage bag, which was tied off and placed on the gurney before the bag was zipped for the last time. Together, the remnants of the bodies would be sent back to the Anatomical Gift Association, where they would be cremated prior to being returned to their families.

Most medical schools choose to honor the sacrifices of the donating individuals when it is all done by hosting a Service of Gratitude. At some institutions, the donors' families are invited; they can meet the group of aspiring physicians and receive thanks in the form of conversation, music, and poetry. While my school did not honor the families in this particular way, we did host a ceremony, wrote poems and letters, and composed musical pieces in remembrance of our cadavers, nonetheless. We swapped our scrubs for blazers, skinny ties, dresses, and heels, and we bowed our heads together in remembrance. Sand-wiched between an opening bugle call and a bagpipe perfor-mance of "Amazing Grace," my classmates shared at the podium how much this experience had changed them. Some of my friends acknowledged their complacency, their desensitization for weeks at a time, brought back to the truth by the realization that they might have been the last to ever hold this person's hand. Some had learned how to confront death without fear, how to salvage and embrace the humanity within themselves, how to appreciate this unconditional gift and honor the donors' legacy by allowing their spirit to live on forever through their own career in medicine.

Leaving the ceremony, I focused on my movements, counting the steps out the door, the time passing second by second, paying close attention to the emotions sweeping over, a gust of cold air confronting me as I left. Like a child walking through the double doors on the last day of school, I knew something significant had happened.

Three months prior to the Service of Gratitude, I entered medical school with a grandiose optimism that each new experi-ence would present itself in a tidy package with a bow on top. Here is a learning experience; here is how you can accomplish it and mature as a physician and scientist: "Slide fifty-two, memo-rize this table on the innervation of each compartment of the lower limb." "Do not put a needle under vertebral body L1; the spinal cord is there. Aim for L4." "Try to sit when you take a patient history; it alters the power dynamic."

When anatomy finally came to an end, I found it disap-pointing that I did not know how to feel. I wanted to believe that I came out a changed person—I am not sure how anybody could not be after going through that—but the tension I experienced was from not yet knowing how, not yet being able to stand back and point to somewhere that I had objectively grown. I am jealous of those who were able to identify tangible takeaways, who changed through this experience and could articulate it so beautifully and publicly.

Was I personally more adept to handle mortality? Did I confront the fact that the pain and suffering I'd witnessed every day for nearly three months would someday introduce itself to me? Did I learn what a *"Netter's"* body should look like? I suppose I could say that I emerged from anatomy with a new set of skills. I probably was a better team player than I was before the start of the course. I could now read the basics of a computerized tomography (CT) scan, and I knew the differences between a T1- and T2-weighted magnetic resonance image (MRI). I had a better understanding of the vasculature of the body, how and where muscles insert to accomplish their actions, but what else came from this gift? What did I gain from it that wasn't entirely selfish? Am I a better person than I was before the first cut?

I wish I could tell my younger self that I was supposed to feel happy for making it out the other side, that this was a rite of passage on the road to becoming a physician and that I'd cleared yet another enormous hurdle. That I could confirm how I was one step closer to achieving my goals. To not feel bad about what I saw and thought and said and did. Or if I could tell myself to feel bad, or even something else entirely, because emotional ambivalence somehow felt worse than the second iteration of disgust, distress, and guilt. Tell me: How is it that, after all this, I could feel so profoundly different yet so wholly unchanged?

3

FIELD REPORT

There are these two young fish swimming along, and they happen to meet an older fish swimming the other way, who nods at them and says, "Morning, boys. How's the water?" And the two young fish swim for a bit, and then eventually one of them looks over at the other and goes, "What the hell's water?"

—David Foster Wallace, "This is Water"

I AWOKE at 3:00 a.m. on my right side with my knees pressed firmly to my chest, a diffuse pain radiating from some unidentifiable hearth within my abdomen. I felt on the verge of bursting from the waist, and in an effort to alleviate the discomfort, I rolled onto my back to look at my bulging stomach. Exploring the outer surface of my midsection with my hands did nothing but confirm these observations. Because every minor movement exacerbated the pain, I remained frozen, face buried in my pillow, squeezing my eyes tighter and tighter until the world went dark.

By 5:00 a.m., the dull roar had grown into a different beast, feasting on my insides and evolving into sharp pangs, implacable, like the waves of high tide crashing within my digestive system. Every few minutes, I could feel my bowels peristalsing in reverse from my intestines up through the pyloric sphincter, into my stomach, and toward my esophagus. My tongue began to water, that stinging, metallic-tasting saliva.

"Run. Go. Now! You can do this."

I sprinted down the hall, my naked feet pounding on the cold hardwood, and a half-digested chicken breast soon came out in dehydrated chunks, falling into the porcelain bowl below. This process repeated itself twice more before sunrise. By the third time, all that remained was saliva and bile. Foamy and sour.

In between dry-heaving episodes, I found myself trying to calm my mind from the bathroom floor by googling anything that could be the cause. Food poisoning. Gallstones. Hepatitis. Appendicitis. Pancreatitis. A few of the lectures I had attended that week touched on abdominal physiology, and I couldn't help but wonder if I was afflicted by any number of the diseases I was studying. I had heard of this before, the infamous "Medical Student Syndrome," a version of hypochondriasis specific to medical trainees. To reject these suspicions, I tried to sleep through the pain a second time, a battle I could not help but lose.

By 8:00 a.m., motivated by fear of the sustained vomiting episodes, I surrendered to professional help. Unable to make the trek across campus to student health, I called an Uber to my appointment. Minutes later, I was face-to-face with a doctor running through the seven descriptors of pain: site, onset, provocation, quality, radiation, severity, and timing. I told him I'd been experiencing pain in my midline stomach since the early morning which had since migrated to the right lower quadrant. I told him about the associated nausea and vomiting and the distension in my abdomen as well. He asked me a few more questions before requesting that I lift my shirt for the physical exam.

As he palpated my abdomen, applying first shallow then deep pressure, I reflected on what it must be like to go into surgery: cold, exposed, vulnerable. It scared me.

"Ouch! That hurts."

"Right here?"

"Ow, yes, there."

"Rebound tenderness in the right lower quadrant."

I knew we were both thinking the same thing. To confirm the diagnosis of appendicitis and rule out any other differential diagnoses, the doctor picked up his landline and scheduled an ultrasound at two that afternoon. As he hung up on radiology, he turned toward me with a surprised look, chuckling as he said, "It is very unusual to obtain an appointment with them the same day."

I laughed too, mainly because I found it unusual that this haste would *not* be expected, provided we both were under the impression that my apparently inflamed appendix could rupture if left untreated for an extended period of time. I was perplexed, also, by his relative lack of urgency given the severity of my symptoms, but I deferred to his expertise and resigned myself to playing the role of the patient, one who waits.

Before I left student health that morning, it was recommended that I have bloodwork drawn, and as I stood up to leave the phlebotomy chair a few minutes later with three new needle holes in my left arm, the nurse commented, "You look terrible."

She wasn't wrong. I had sweat through my clothes, my hair was matted to my head from the night before, I was pretty sure part of my dinner was on my shirt, and I reeked of vomit. When the appointment concluded, I had nowhere else to be, so I limped across the hospital to the radiology department and informed them that I was there for my appointment in three hours. To my surprise, the ultrasound tech called me in early, and from the dark of the procedure room, she pulsed sound waves throughout my abdomen, taking images of the vibrations that returned to the monitor. I managed to fall asleep multiple times during the imaging session, awoken an equal number of times by a tender nudge to roll onto my side. When I left the room, the tech informed me that the results would be posted within the hour. I decided to wait at the hospital in case I needed to be rushed into emergent surgery. And because it hurt to move.

Three hours passed until I finally received a call with the results. The person on the other end of the line informed me that the ultrasound found "free fluid" pooling in my abdomen along with "prominent bowel loops." Negative for gallstones. Negative for appendicitis. I was not entirely sure what to make of these findings and neither was the voice on the other end of the line, who ultimately recommended further evaluation with a "cat scan." We scheduled the appointment for 7:30 that same evening. He told me that, between now and then, I could eat for the first time that day, and clearly altered from sleep deprivation, I decided to purchase a hamburger from the hospital vending machine and camp there until the evening. In the interim, I reviewed the lectures I had missed from earlier in the day.

At 6:30 p.m. back at radiology, I was greeted in the waiting room with 930 mL of diluted contrast. The receptionist handed me a packet of Crystal Light to help the iodine-laced mixed drink taste less bitter. I was told I had an hour to drink it in its entirety. She told me to try not to throw it up and I complied. In between sips, I checked my Instagram feed and the News app and back again like I had a hundred times that day, welcoming the flurry of incoming information as it populated the rectangle in my hand. An hour later, there was still no sign of the radiologist, and as I had drunk all the contrast, I again began to feel on the verge of bursting, this time not from pain but from the urgent need to urinate. Unsure if I was allowed to relieve myself without ruining the findings of the upcoming CT, and being the only person in the waiting room at that hour of the night, I paced feverishly until the front desk assistant returned from break. During a respite from an argument with her bank over the status of her student loans, she informed me I was allowed to use the restroom. I proceeded to pee for what must have been ninety uninterrupted seconds and forgave all those who had transgressed against me. Life was suddenly that much better.

Two hours after my arrival and another hour after my scheduled appointment, I queried the front desk assistant about the delay, and a moment later, the radiologist burst into the waiting room, where I was the only patron, and called me through the double doors. In the back room, I was ushered to the large, metallic donut where I was positioned supine and inserted halfway into the machine. I was informed that a tech would place an IV into my arm to help the contrast light up on the imaging software, providing a clear picture of my internal organs. As the machine noisily enveloped me, a chemical was injected into my bloodstream. Immediately, I felt it mobilize. It started with a warmth in my right arm, the median cubital vein, quickly traveling to my chest, then inside my atria and ventricles. With each exhale, I could taste my silvery breath escaping into the room.

I mumbled to myself, "Please don't throw up. Keep it together."

With each beat of my heart, the heat radiated further and further to the periphery before aggressively concentrating in my groin.

"Am I peeing myself?"

"No," the tech assured me.

A giant scanner circled overhead and zoomed over me. An automated voice called out, "Breathe in. Hold."

At 9:15 p.m., I was told they were finished and that the results would be up in two days.

As I made my way home that night, I reflected on how extraordinarily unsatisfying it had been to be on the other side of the patient-provider relationship. The most frustrating part of the day was not even necessarily the abdominal pain, but mostly the feeling of being lost. With each visit to the urgent care, the ultrasound room, and the radiologist, I had hoped that somebody would have been able to absolve me of this feeling and put me at ease. For over twelve hours, though, I'd bounced between departments and waiting rooms, confused. Of all people, I recognized that, in this setting, I was in a position of relative privilege. I was insured. I was generally aware of what could potentially be happening to my body, the relative urgency of those possible scenarios, and although I was more familiar with the demands of a busy clinic, even I had no idea what was occurring behind the scenes, and my caretakers did little with their opportunities to assuage my fears.

I can't imagine a field that exists with a greater degree of informational asymmetry than medicine. I can think of disciplines like law or tax accounting where there is so much nuance that nearly everyone does, in fact, rely on the existence of specialists to act as interpreters to make informed choices, but there is something inherently more intimate about the gatekeepers of personal health information whereby a patient relies entirely on a doctor's professional opinion to inform their own. Because of this, patients are at the whim of another's ability and desire to enlighten. As a concept, this is fascinating in a scream-into-the-void kind of way.

In college, I worked in a lab researching neuroanatomical connections in the primate motor cortex. The nature of my research required the study of animal models, specifically nonhuman primates like squirrel monkeys and macaques. Macaques are a large species of primate that are susceptible to contagious bacteria and viruses, such as hepatitis B virus and tuberculosis, which can spread across species to humans. For these reasons, every few months while I worked there, I was required to undergo blood tests and medical screenings to ensure the safety of us students as well as the expensive lab animals helping scientists revolutionize our concept of the primate central nervous system.

For over two years, I regularly scheduled these screening appointments with the same physician. For two years we would have the same conversation:

"Where are you from?"

"Atlanta."

"Atlanta! I have a daughter in Sandy Springs."

"No kidding, that's not too far away from me."

This is a conversation we had on at least four separate occasions, and each time she didn't remember me, for right or wrong, I questioned how much she cared about my wellbeing. I am aware that she has seen hundreds if not thousands of patients in her career. I know she is trying to make small talk, an attempt to get to know me or to cut the awkward tension in an otherwise quiet room. While the thought was there, the fact remained that the execution was botched not once but on multiple occasions. Unfortunately for her, intent does not change a patient's interpretation of the interaction. She's a bad listener. She's forgetful. Just like my doctors at student health and radiology who lacked urgency. Or punctuality. Or empathy. Or attention to detail. It didn't matter to me, the patient, if they had my best interests in mind because I could not directly observe that goal in action.

Four days, three unreturned emails, and two worried calls from my mother later, I was finally informed that my results were posted. I logged into my online health portal and was greeted by the following header: "22-year-old female with abdominal pain, nausea, vomiting."

Other than learning that my gender had been reassigned, the findings were threefold:

1) *There are a few mildly prominent lymph nodes within the lower right quadrant.*

2) *There is abnormally increased mucosal enhancement and circumferential wall thickening involving the distal ileum, with associated mesenteric vascular engorgement. No evidence of bowel obstruction.*

3) *Left L5 pars defect, which may be congenital.*

> *Although these findings are nonspecific and could*
> *represent a terminal ileitis of any etiology, this*
> *appearance is suspicious for Crohn's disease.*

Crohn's disease? I decided to schedule a consultation with a gastroenterologist as soon as possible. The scheduling assistant informed me that the earliest they could see me was four weeks from then, and I booked it without thinking twice. In the time spent waiting for my appointment, I experienced two other similar, near-paralyzing episodes, each time choosing not to go into the hospital, preferring to risk it and wait it out until the pain subsided, as it had before.

At the specialist's office one month later, I was called into the clinic early for my appointment, where my vitals were taken:

Heart rate: 61 beats per minute

Blood pressure: 115/57

"Diastolic is low," the nurse muttered to herself before shepherding me into a nearby room.

A few minutes later, the specialist walked through the door. She was tall and slim, brunette, with a soft but self-assured voice.

She shook my hand and asked me to take a seat next to her while she fired up the computer. In a matter-of-fact tone, she wasted no time telling me she agreed with the radiologist in believing that I could be suffering from either an acute ileitis or Crohn's disease. It could have been her demeanor, how she noticed the badge clipped to my belt and asked about my classwork, or how she addressed all my questions and even let me see the images of my CT, but I felt safer under her care. We concluded the appointment with her recommending a colonoscopy to better visualize my bowels and obtain samples for the pathology lab, and I walked out of her office after sched-uling the procedure for ten days later.

As I walked down the steps with the Safari browser pulled up on three separate tabs (one with the Wikipedia page for Crohn's disease, another with treatment options on WebMD, and a third with a Google search for symptoms and treatment side effects), a text informed me that my urgent care visit a month ago had racked up a bill of over $12,000. With three zeroes.

Over the next few days, I would've been lying if I said I wasn't terrified to look more into Crohn's disease. My inaction stemmed more from fear than a lack of curiosity—I was not yet ready to hear bad news, and the longer I ignored my fate, the longer I could delay it. Of course, invariably, this logic is flawed, but I figured I could try to live my life in ignorant bliss until the diagnosis was confirmed.

For the two days prior to the colonoscopy, my prep work began. First, I learned that I was restricted to a clear liquid diet, allowed to eat only applesauce, popsicles, and chicken broth. Per the instructions, at noon, I was to take two tablets of Dulcolax.

At 1:15 p.m. that same day, I went to my afternoon classes, where I was scheduled to conduct my first patient interview in the clinical skills curriculum. My role was to practice taking a history of present illness (HPI), which involved introducing myself to a patient actor and asking questions about what brought them into "clinic" for the day. When I knocked on the door, I suddenly felt the urgent need to defecate. I have no idea how I performed during this exam, but when the session ended, I ran out of the room as fast as I could, clenching my anal sphincter to the best of my ability, hoping to God that those tiny muscles I had seen in the cadaver lab did not run out of adenosine triphosphate (ATP) or calcium. When I made it safely to the bathroom, the gates opened in a violent bout of diarrhea, gates that would not close for the next forty-eight hours.

"At 6:00 p.m., take half of the bottle of Miralax." Sweet Jesus. I complied and poured seven servings of laxatives into a cocktail of blue Powerade. At the point of making this mixture, morale was admittedly low, and my stool had already reached the consistency of what the brochure described as the ideal "yellow liquid."

The next day at 12:00 p.m., I was instructed to, again, drink seven servings of laxatives.

"DO NOT SKIP THIS STEP," it read.

Against my better judgment, I skipped the step because I was hungry and angry and dehydrated and hadn't stopped shitting yellow water since the early afternoon of the previous day. At 3:00 p.m., I arrived at my appointment with two slices of Papa Johns in a to-go container as my reward for when I eventually made it out of the procedure.

"When was the last time you ate?"

"I had apple sauce this morning."

"Did you complete the regimen?"

"Yes," I lied, knowing they could figuratively see through me and would literally see in me soon enough. I decided it was better to delay the shame and make them discover the evidence instead of outing myself then and there.

At 5:30 p.m., I was injected with a mild sedative and greeted in the back room by my doc, a nurse, and a fellow. As they commenced, I could feel air being injected into my rectum at a PSI of twenty-eight, I guessed, expanding the lumen of my digestive tract as it cleared space for the insertion of a probe. As the air traversed the turns of my large intestine and the scope advanced, I heard an acceleration of rhythmic beeping, and the monitor tracking my heart rate jumped from 58 to 85. Throughout the procedure, I watched on the tiny television as the camera explored my insides, pausing only to take a few biopsies from the walls of my intestine.

A week later, my gastroenterologist went through the images from the procedure. In one panel, she pointed out a collection of polyps she had excised and sent off to pathology. In another, I saw a transverse colon full of yellow fecal matter with the label "Poor Prep." My face turned red because I knew this would come back to haunt me, though this time, she let me off the hook and skipped over the image. In the third and final panel, she pointed to a section of inflamed tissue.

"So, this is the ileocecal valve. As you can see, the inflammation is so extensive that I couldn't get the probe through. This is indicative of Crohn's disease."

I mostly stopped listening from there, but my ears perked up when she told me I had a few treatment options. The presentation of my Crohn's disease was what she described as "stricturing," meaning that, because the disease had been present for so long, the ileocecal valve was all but impenetrable. Over time, presumably many years of indolent inflammation, it had been reduced to a fibrotic pinhole instead of a flexible tube, and the symptoms which initially brought me to care were caused by this ring of scar tissue, as various foods simply could not get past the stricture and would cause what she called "self-resolving obstructive episodes." This, evidently, was a more severe type of Crohn's, one that was not treatable with the anti-inflammatory medications I had researched online days prior and had prepared myself to push for her to prescribe.

She explained to me that I could, however, start on an expensive class of biologic drugs—anti-tumor necrosis factor alpha (TNF) medications—which target hyperactive inflammatory messengers in my digestive system. These drugs are directly administered via the blood, so as to avoid degradation by the harsh stomach enzymes. My treatment options effectively boiled down to an IV infusion lasting an hour in the hospital once every eight weeks or self-administered injections every two weeks. I told my doctor that this was a lot of information to process and that I wanted to discuss it with my family.

When I went home, I again found it difficult to overcome the activation energy, struggling to open my computer and research the risks and benefits of each option. It was not that I didn't want to do the research on my own. I actually really wanted to but, quite frankly, I feared what I would find. What I didn't want to hear was that Crohn's disease was a type of inflammatory bowel disease that was caused by an overactive immune response, often targeting the end of the small intestine. Common symptoms included weight loss, abdominal pain, and diarrhea, and it was associated with serious complications, some of which I was already familiar with (bowel obstructions) and some of which I was only beginning to learn about. I didn't want to learn that there were serious side effects to the drugs recommended, like an increased risk of infection and cancer, or that there was no cure for Crohn's or an end to treatment once initiated, that whatever I chose would likely be a lifelong decision, or at least until my body started to recognize the medication and reject it and I would have to find a new treatment.

Crohn's isn't exactly the most serious disease out there, but I knew it could be life-altering. In my Googling, I found studies reporting that 75 percent of Crohn's patients eventually had to get surgery, often within five years of diagnosis, sometimes to excise a stricture or fistula, other times to make an ileostomy bag. Even after surgery, in many of these cases, the disease recurred in a different part of the intestine. If left untreated, people could develop debilitating fistulas, worsening obstructive episodes, and painful skin conditions associated with autoimmune overdrive. None of that sounded appealing. Then again, injecting myself with an immunosuppressant every other week for the rest of my life wasn't ideal either, especially given my career mandated working in a hospital setting with infectious diseases floating in the air and settling on every hard surface.

Eventually, I decided on the self-administered treatment option called Humira, or the highest-grossing biologic ever made. My hands were tied, and I wanted to get better, so I submitted and hoped my future could be like those oversaturated commercials playing at the halftimes of every other college football game. A mother chasing after her child in a generic field of lilies. A stock shot of a grandpa walking out of a porta-potty at a 12U soccer game and never looking back. A youngish forty-something strolling down Main Street to uplifting piano music. I thought if I could just regain this level of normalcy, then I could be satisfied with this decision.

Shortly after the new year, a package arrived at my front door. I brought it inside and cut the tape overlying the opposed edges. Once it was open, I pulled the lid off a Styrofoam cooler and removed a freezer pack sitting snugly inside. I unzipped the Ziplock baggie housing the smaller, perforated cardboard box and tore into it. Inside were two pens, one of which I placed in the refrigerator for safekeeping, the other of which I left at room temperature on my granite countertop to equilibrate with the outside environment. After thirty minutes, I grabbed the purple cylinder and followed the instructions from an application I had downloaded on my phone just moments before, first using an alcohol wipe to disinfect a small circle on my inner left thigh, then sequentially removing the caps on both sides of the pen. I pressed its open end against my leg, hesitated for a split second, and with a deep breath, pushed the button on the end, releasing the spring-loaded mechanism and sending the needle sliding effortlessly through my skin. After an audible squirt informed me that the medication had been released, I withdrew the pen, and blood soon began oozing out, following the curve of my leg as it trailed downward.

This diagnosis does not define who I am. I know that life goes on, but it would be a green assertion to say that things would stay the same when not a day goes by where I don't think about how this has affected me, and not a meal passes where I can choose to ignore this condition. While a diagnosis of Crohn's disease certainly is not the worst thing that has ever happened to anybody, and it almost seems trivial in comparison to other health or personal tragedies, the dietary restrictions I place on myself every day, the biweekly plunges into my thigh, the blood draws and colonoscopy checkups and MRIs and obstructive episodes I've experienced despite all these measures serve as mementos of how my body has betrayed me. They are daily reminders of the fragility of health and mere existence and of the quality-adjusted life years (QALYs) I have lost. My story is not even close to over. I have no idea where it is going, and the loss of control frightens me.

I would never choose to do it in this way, but I suppose this chronic illness experience has allowed me to better empathize with future patients. I have been forced to walk a mile in the shoes of others, and I've learned so much about doctoring from this side of the room. I've absorbed from providers—both those who have treated me right and the ones whom I've despised—which behaviors I hope to emulate one day and which I seek to avoid. Above all else, I have learned that, when it comes down to it, health is a luxury. Most people live their lives not considering that this could all go away in an instant. They are the lucky ones, and looking back from here, I had more than two decades of luck. I woke up every morning and felt young and invincible. I worked out and thought about what foods I put in my body; I washed my hands and got my flu shot. I thought I was doing everything right, and to an extent, these behaviors protected, and continue to protect me, from a lot of preventable disease down the road.

For other diseases, one day the outlook is brilliant and the next it's upside down. Cancer. Lupus. Crohn's disease. Nobody ever suspects it's going to be them until it is, and it always seems to come at the most unpredictable and inconvenient of times. Disease cares not about limits and steals volition. It takes away agency and has no regrets about it, forcing us to change our status quo to its whims, to become chronically dependent on something outside of ourselves all while it slowly chips away at our defenses.

Father Time is unrelenting and Mother Nature can only be so generous, but in this life, where there are never enough answers, we must not live in fear of what comes next. Bad things happen and people die and nothing ever really makes sense. But when the shit hits the fan, we have a choice to collapse under the weight of this madness or face our problems head on—to recognize the inherent value of our present state of being, how precious and fleeting and random all of this is around us.

4

DANCE LESSONS

Tedious repetitions of routine actions make us great.

—Mike Tomlin

MOST THURSDAY AFTERNOONS during MS1 were dedicated to the clinical skills curriculum. The premise was actually quite simple: during an appointment, a physician must ask dozens of questions to accurately diagnose a condition, and medical students must eventually figure out how to do this efficiently and effectively. In practice, however, the questions doctors pose become much more deliberate as a visit progresses. To practice this, one must get comfortable with the act of performing a history and physical exam, the H&P.

We are taught this process in medical school and attempt to familiarize ourselves with memory hooks of our own (e.g.,

SOCRATES, VINDICATE, PQRST, etc.) such that we do not miss any key components of this information gathering step.

Site (Where is the pain?)
Onset (What were they doing when the symptoms started?)
Character (What does it feel like?)
Radiate (Does the pain go elsewhere?)
Associate (Are there any other associated symptoms?)
Time (How long have the symptoms been present?)
Exacerbate/alleviate (What makes it better or worse?)
Severity (How severe are the symptoms on a scale of 1–10?)

We were also taught in this course how to speak like a doctor: "I am going to *feel* for your pulse" was replaced with our new "ICE" mnemonic, short for inspect, check, and examine. "I am going to *check* for your pulse," which evidently had a subtle effect on the subconscious of a patient who did not want to be felt, rather checked, by their doctor. We learned to not "question stack" with yes or no queries but to instead lead with open ended questions: "Is the pain burning? Pounding? Stabbing?" became "Describe your pain for me." We were instructed how to properly position our hands when performing the physical exam. I learned that all these tiny details that seemed natural to doctors were at one point taught to them and taught in the most excruciating detail: "Nondominant hand on top of dominant hand." "Light pressure, then deep for the abdominal exam." "Auscultate for bowel sounds *before* palpating." "Hold your breath with the patient when you listen for carotid pulses."

The words doctors use, the way they address individuals, the orientation of their stethoscopes, the side of the patient they stand on, how they enter a room and adjust a drape, the questions they ask, and even the so-called neutral utterances they use to fill the time between sentences were all built into lectures. "I see." "Hmm." "I'm so sorry to hear that." Talk before touch is a staple of the clinical skills curriculum, and the art of being a physician is as much a formula as it is improvisation.

Clinical skills days were largely spent in groups of four with one "Standardized Patient," or SP for short, assigned to us. SPs were actors paid by the medical school to personify a specific medical problem which we, the medical students, were to discover in brief, timed interactions. For the most part, they were excellent resources at our disposal, though across the board, I found that they were vehemently invested in their "roles," as if they were auditioning for the next big summer flick and their ability to pay rent depended on whether they got the part: masked facies became a perversion of Parkinson's disease. An SP feigning depression talked at a speed of fifteen words-per-minute. A case of domestic abuse was hidden in five layers of questioning and a fake bruise painted in make-up on their chest. We often joked that these actors took their roles so seriously that, if we told them to breathe in and hold their breath, they wouldn't resume breathing until we gave them permission.

Prior to my first SP interaction, I anticipated that the "appointment" would go something like the way I had practiced on my roommates, except instead of interviewing and examining the patient on my kitchen table, the visit would be held in a pretend clinic in the basement of our academic building, with cameras recording our every move.

Test days typically followed the same script. We were presented with a prompt such as: "Chris presents with a chief complaint of shortness of breath." We would then have twenty minutes to perform the H&P, and afterward, the curtain would come down and the SP would ask us what we thought went well and what could have gone more smoothly, and with any time remaining, we would role-play a part of the visit that could have been improved. Most of the time, their feedback was helpful, providing alternative ways I could have inquired about sensitive subjects or family members passing away, but other times, I received more bogus criticism about how I lost points on the extremity exam for failing to look at the skin on the back of their elbow for possible malignant melanoma.

After these sessions, we were required to watch recordings of ourselves interviewing the SPs in order to learn our own quirks, the filler words we liked to use, how we shifted in our seats when we sat down, the way we fidgeted with our pens at uncomfortable moments.

On one of these fated afternoons, we were scheduled to learn the male genitourinary exam. This was important for evaluating sexually transmitted infections, testicular masses, and torsion, for instance, and involved combing through pubic hair, looking for lesions on the penis, checking for swollen lymph nodes, and performing an inguinal hernia check. Of course, given the sensitive nature of the exam, we were all apprehensive, which was not alleviated when the SP disrobed, and we were met with the largest penis to which we had ever borne witness. This was verified in multiple conversations after the session concluded: a certified show-er.

As of this incident, I had seen at least six flaccid penises in my life: my own, my dad's when I was a kid, my baseball teammate's on accident, and those of a few random older gentlemen walking shamelessly around the locker rooms of Life Time. Though I judged from this admittedly small sample size, this one took the cake by at least two standard deviations. Quite frankly alarmed by this finding, I stood off to the side while my female colleague took the first pass for us.

The SP began, "OK, so to start, you're going to want to put on gloves. You'll then ask the patient to take off his pants, which I have already done for you. Any idea what's next?"

My classmate timidly inched forward and responded, "Alright sir, I'm going to start with the visual exam. I do not see any obvious lesions."

As we were taught, she checked all surfaces of the penis, making sure to look inside its accompanying orifice for any signs of infection or drainage.

"Next, I am going to use the pads of my fingers to check for any swelling of your lymph nodes. There are two chains that run along on each side of your groin that I will be inspecting."

Just as she said, she made small circles using her hands to check for any lymphadenopathy which might suggest infection or cancer.

"Next, for any other patient, I would say 'I am going to examine your pubic hair,' but because you have none, I think this will suffice."

She proceeded to mime out what she would have done had the patient had pubic hair. Employing the index and middle fingers of both hands, she pretended to sift around looking for hidden cuts and sores.

At this moment, the SP reached his hand out and interjected, "Alright, I'm going to stop you there. Your face is getting really close to my penis ..."

———

Even having had no background in medicine prior to entering medical school, it was no surprise to me that being a doctor would be full of challenging interpersonal interactions. I think that medical educators realize that their students are not inherently born with these skills, and for this reason, we practice them in school.

A few times each quarter, we had clinical skills sessions dedicated to, for instance, shared decision-making: "the difficult patient," dealing with drug-seeking behavior, and who could forget, delivering bad news. These sessions included a student as the doctor, the patient played by an SP, and an audience, usually the other three group members, who did not actively have a role. As a conflict-averse personality who was also more reserved at baseline, I always dreaded these sessions. They made me extraordinarily uncomfortable. While we rotated on a set agenda, I much preferred to watch.

One afternoon, we were told that a patient who smoked a pack of cigarettes daily for her entire adult life was coming into clinic. She had been experiencing a cough for a few months and had received a chest X-ray a week ago. She was now back in the office for the interpretation, which showed unequivocal lung cancer. The objective was to deliver the news.

Thankfully, God smiled on me that day and it was not my turn to go, so I lined up in a chair with two other classmates on the wall of the patient room. Situated on the other side next to a computer and a small desk was our SP for the afternoon. Our fourth, the "doctor" for the day, knocked before entering.

He began, "Hello, Mrs. Smith. Thank you for coming in today. It's nice to see you again."

Mrs. Smith replied, "Yes, doctor it's good to see you too."

"How are you feeling?"

"I'm doing alright. I'm just really nervous about the results. I've been thinking about them all week."

"You know, that response is completely reasonable, and if nothing else, we should be able to provide you some answers today. Along those lines, I am sorry to say that I do have some tough news to deliver. I looked at your chest X-ray, and it shows a mass in your left lung. We will likely need a biopsy to know what it is for certain, but I am afraid it is lung cancer."

Following the delivery of this news, the patient burst into tears, giant crocodile tears, right on cue, saying, "Ugh, I knew that's what it was going to be. It's because of the smoking, isn't it? I hate myself. I've been smoking for thirty years. I knew this was going to happen."

My classmate rebuffed, "I know this is hard to hear, but Mrs. Smith, what's done is done. There is no sense in placing blame anywhere. We just have to get through this together."

She challenged, "I'm DYING for God's sake!" Her screams echoed throughout the clinic. "How can you say that?!?"

There was a long pause as he contemplated what to say next before trailing off, "Well, technically we're all dying ..."

———

When we were not interviewing SPs, once a week in the clinical skills curriculum, we were released into the wild to interview a real patient. Our advisor would give us a list of patients with varying chief complaints, and we would venture over to the hospital and ask for permission to enter. Most patients were understanding and often humored me as I fumbled through a disorganized H&P. This was our experience with the wards as MSIs, distilled into these practice sessions on real people. The contrast between this and the SP encounter could not be more obvious.

A full H&P includes, of course, the history of presenting illness (HPI), where we inquire about a patient's current symptoms. To complete the picture, though, there are numerous other pertinent details which often are not offered by a patient, as they might not think it is related to their presenting condition. For example, a patient with fatigue and infectious symptoms might not appreciate that their blood sugar could be a cause, but knowing they have a medical history of diabetes can offer insight into their condition as well as trigger concern for potential complications if left untreated.

In addition to the medical history, we are instructed to inquire about relevant surgical history, medications, allergies, and social history, including alcohol, tobacco, and drug use. We scour the medical record for laboratory abnormalities and peruse their imaging for positive findings on CT scans and X-rays.

During the SP encounter, we are encouraged to complete the entirety of the H&P, and we are docked for failing to complete a section. In real life, however, the H&P is much more nuanced. For a patient who has just broken their ankle, inquiring about the number of sexual partners they had in the past year is not relevant, and instead, might be seen as intrusive. For a ninety-year-old patient presenting to the emergency department (ED) with chest pain, beginning an encounter by asking about their pronouns might cause confusion instead of understanding.

At this point in my first year, I had learned that so much

about medicine, from the structure of the patient interview to management decisions, could be algorithmic, and in SP encounters, it often felt like I was following a script because, in actuality, I was. The song and dance of running a patient encounter had to be memorized so I would not be distracted by red herrings or succumb to any number of cognitive biases. The reality of being on the wards instead of in the clinical skills classroom was that human experiences were constantly showing me how quickly these algorithms could fall apart, that when I ask somebody about their drug use history and they say "meth and fentanyl," I am supposed to make a mental note and continue with the interview. Sometime later, instead of placing my stethoscope on the chest of somebody with a normal cardiac physiology, I will hear and diagnose a murmur for the first time. Suddenly, the music will stop and my dance partner will be gone, and I will understand that using the script as a framework to move past that discomfort is partially what separates a medical student from a practicing physician.

One day, a classmate shared a story from one of these interactions during MSI. She was interviewing an older man who was admitted for a chronic obstructive pulmonary disease (COPD) exacerbation. In her history-taking, she could not help but feel sorry for this man, who had kindly agreed to be interviewed but was struggling to breathe while he answered her questions. She learned that he had a family back home waiting for him upon his discharge from the hospital and that he enjoyed playing chess in his free time. In the social history, she discovered that he had spent an extended time in prison. Reflexively, she asked him what he did, to which he responded, "rape."

Her mind raced with questions like: "How could you do such

a disgusting thing?" "What kind of monster are you?" "What gives you the right to steal the innocence from another person, to saddle them with a lifetime of trauma, fear, guilt, and anger?"

She then took a moment to collect her thoughts before asking the only question she could think to ask: "Do you have any allergies?"

5

A YEAR IN REVIEW

I believe every human has a finite number of heartbeats. I don't intend to waste any of mine.

—Neil Armstrong

THE LIFE of a student is one of many beginnings and endings, of orientations and commencements, of normalcy in cycles. At the beginning of each year, we start something undifferentiated before realizing a comfort zone only to lose it again. We must then find a balance once more, as we have done annually for the past two decades. In a sense, change is our constant.

This time, I completed the 17th grade, and yet again I found myself at these crossroads, a feeling that was so familiar. I looked around and knew there was so much to be done, more work and investment and studying on the horizon. I saw my parents brimming with pride for another year checked off the

list. I saw a winding road that I could take back to my hometown where time stands still, back to my friends who would be
there starting new jobs and new lives, raising families of their
own. I looked behind me and could now see all that I'd
traversed.

The first year of medical school was a whirlwind, but overall,
it was better than I could have expected. I somehow survived
drinking from the firehose without drowning entirely, serially
cramming for exams in anatomy and physiology, biochemistry,
health equity, immunology, and statistics. While we covered a
remarkable amount of information and perhaps more in life
experience, at the same time, I find it challenging to rattle off a
list of specific examples. Learning moments continued to
present longitudinally instead of anecdotally.

Of course, in what was left of my free time outside of class, I
continued conducting research with my mentors. I continued
going to clinical skills sessions, where I was taught how to confi-
dently ask a patient about their sexually transmitted infections,
alcohol and drug use history, and family history of cancers,
autoimmune conditions, and heart disease. I learned how to
perform the breast exam on a real-life boob and how to administer a prostate exam by sticking my finger into the real-life b-
hole of another man. I went to microbiology, where I learned
about bacteria and parasites and fungi, and I was introduced in
pathology to anything and everything that could go wrong in the
human body.

As a group, we also welcomed our collective new seats at the
table in broader conversations about healthcare access. We
joined clubs, organized rallies for Deferred Action for Childhood Arrivals (DACA), championed research on gun violence
prevention, and spent some of our free time participating in

activities outside of medicine that we cared about, as one is ought to do during MSI.

The novel thing about extracurricular activities in medical school is that students are free to explore their passions, a dynamic so surprisingly and remarkably different from every other period in my past. In high school, my counselors and teachers all seemed to know what colleges wanted out of their prospective students. They loved community service, I was told, and like a chameleon, I took on the form of who I thought they wanted me to become. The system was designed to create community servants, student government presidents, Habitat for Humanity treasurers, and bike drive organizers, all for this grand illusion that I was not just dedicated but *drawn to* the greater good. There was nothing wrong with this approach, and of course, I wanted to leave the world a better place than it was when I arrived. In all likelihood, these activities contributed to making me a better person, allowing me to give back to those less fortunate and generally to be a contributing member of society. By default, though, I traded potential moments of self-discovery, never allowing myself to even glance at the more whimsical flyers that adorned the stairwells (who the hell had time for Anime club?), for this appearance of making a difference. I played the game, and the system created a cookie-cutter college candidate. Luckily for me, it panned out, and with each success story, the cycle repeats, further ingraining itself with each new candidate.

In college, when I decided I would be premed, I heard medical schools would be watching my every move. The pressure intensified. I felt the need to be even more calculated about what I did, to create what my advisors called a "common thread" through my application that told a compelling story addressing the question of "why medicine?" I ended up teaching math to elementary-aged children for two spring breaks. I coached a youth baseball team, and I gave golf lessons to kids across town. I enjoyed teaching and mentorship—that was the message I crafted. If sports were thrown in, then that was a bonus because I liked that, too. My research was on the motor cortex. I dedicated a lot of hours to a pediatrics community outreach project. I volunteered at my university's free clinic. Check, check, check.

Medical school is a completely different experience. Residency programs, for the most part, don't care about what an applicant does in their free time. Get the grades and crush the boards and all is well. So, what students do in their free time in medical school from there is up to them. There aren't necessarily club members, at least at my medical school, only club leaders, and so the leaders of the clubs organize events every quarter for anybody to sign up and participate in. It's a fascinating dichotomy shift. I could have been as involved or uninvolved as I liked. I could explore new events and service opportunities. I could push for diversity in surgery as a leader of the interest group, promote childhood literacy as an ambassador for Reach Out and Read, join the Wellness Committee and plan parties for my fellow classmates. I could do all of this while signing up for five different intramural teams, including inner tube water polo and broomball, and exploring different specialties by attending a "Psychology of Gambling" talk and an otolaryngology Q&A. And this was exactly what I did.

Research is the same story. I came into college having absolutely no clue about research as a concept. The only thing I knew was that, if I was going to be premed, I should probably do it. I joined the first project I was offered in an attempt to figure out what the heck it was. My journey from clinical research (focused on clinical outcomes) to basic science (understanding how the world works) to translational (integrating the two), while circuitous, allowed me to gain exposure to a variety of fields and technical skills and, eventually, to figure out my interests, which I would be free to explore as a medical student. While research in the first year of medical school is by no means required, I started on several projects investigating a variety of surgical outcomes, eventually posing my own hypotheses and designing studies exploring questions to which I really wanted to know the answers. I had earned the autonomy.

Other than that, I just have these nonspecific memories of the daily grind, and to be honest, it's not really memories, it's memories of having a memory. I know I lived through first year, but the details are washed out, an acetone bath of nostalgia with a sprinkle of post-traumatic stress disorder. But I did survive the longest academic year of my life, lasting from August to June, and for all the weird encounters and happenstance of that year, MS1 was overwhelmingly positive. I felt that I finally had the chance to thrive both academically and socially.

As the summer wound to a close, at the conclusion of the summer research program between MS1 and MS2, I stood at those crossroads again, staring at what was ahead. Honestly, from there, the future appeared bleak. Pathophysiology looked like a road full of potholes and the upcoming board exams a gigantic storm cloud. I saw it in the second years who were gearing up for study block, telling us to cherish what we had every chance we got. I saw it in the absence of the third years, whom we affectionately called "unicorns" if we ever saw them because they basically lived in the hospital. I saw it in the fourth years in all their infinite wisdom, telling us to hold onto what we had because it flew by.

———

Around New Year's every year, Google publishes a video called "Year in Search." In these clips, they feature a Google search bar with a theme typed into the search engine. What follows is a seamless transition to images spliced from various events in the year. 2017 highlighted the escalating conflict with North Korea, Trump's inauguration, hurricanes, the refugee crisis, the mass shooting in Las Vegas, the Women's March, the solar eclipse, and the "Me Too" movement. Each somehow managed to elicit the same reaction: "Wow, did you remember when that happened?" "That was this year?" "We are living through history." They are moments that made us cry, made us angry, gave us hope, and offered us inspiration.

Watching these reviews, I can't help but think in terms of my own life and ponder for a moment what the review would look like from my first year in medical school. There would be scenes from the scavenger hunt during orientation where I reenacted the duel from Hamilton with a new friend. The welcome barbecue where I sat on Promontory Point in the middle of August, freezing as twenty-mile-per-hour winds cut through my clothing. My birthday party when nearly all eighty-eight members of my class squeezed into my apartment in celebration of both me and finishing the lower limb module of anatomy. There would be a montage of me scavenging for free food at every lunch talk. A clip dedicated to studying in the sunroom of my apartment, every now and then waving through the window at my neighbor in the adjacent apartment who also liked to study in her sunroom. Hospital visits. Patient interviews. Intermittent shots of phone calls to my parents, stressing out about the next exam.

It would feature long conversations with Jason, Ryan, and Russell about relationships, friendships, and the state of American healthcare. Games of slap cup, king's cup, and flip cup. Settlers of Catan and Monopoly Deal. It would end with a pan over of Friendsgiving and a hungover ride to the airport, and maybe that's the best way I can describe the experience of medical school through MS1: I was exhausted from the experiences constantly being thrown at me, but I continued to indulge, despite the effect that it had on my body, because I would rather be hungover from medical school than clearheaded the next day from doing anything else with my life.

MS2

6

_____

STEP BY STEP

And what kind of citizen
does this thought make me, quivering and flummoxed
by contradictory impulses: to give a speech on empathy
or fling my double latte
across his back windshield, though who knows what
he might do then. He's stuck in traffic and pretends
I'm not watching him looking
in my direction, and people passing doubtless think who is
this idiot fulminating to himself,
or probably they don't;
they've got trouble of their own

—Mark Doty, "Citizens"

THE DAYS of second year were long, but the year flew by. In the
fall, we came back from vacation bright-eyed and bushy-tailed,

refreshed and ready to begin again. Much like the first year's end, the second's early days were filled with an appetite for learning and broad-spectrum optimism.

Soon after our arrival, we hit the ground running. In pharmacology, my cohort and I were required to learn about the over 200 different medication classes used to remedy a number of maladies, each with their associated mechanisms of action and related side effect profiles. Because drug names were comprised of syllables that *seem* entirely random (e.g., ketorolac, carbamazepine, escitalopram), pharmacology at this level is often likened to learning a new language—nobody is born knowing that words ending with the suffix -alol were beta blockers, -olam were benzodiazepines, or -statin were HMG-CoA reductase inhibitors, but before the leaves were off the trees, the new language's intricacies had slowly become second nature. By the advent of winter, the groundwork had officially been laid. We had passed microbiology, immunology, neurobiology, and pharmacology. We had developed a mastery of our new tongue and began to flex this knowledge with our professors and peers, localizing lesions on our fake patients and initiating empiric antibiotics in class discussion sections. All of this led to the capstone course of the preclinical years, Clinical Pathophysiology and Therapeutics (CPP&T).

CPP&T tested the synthesis of all previously acquired knowledge with the diagnosis and management of actual human disease. For six months, we trudged our way through each organ system (heme, vasculature, heart, lungs, gastrointestinal, exocrine, endocrine, renal, reproductive, breast, nervous, musculoskeletal, and skin), learning as we went the minutiae of each disease and how it riddled the body, which populations were most at risk, and the downstream effects of treated and untreated disease.

In order to comb through all of this material in a timely manner, CPP&T lectures started every day at 8:00 a.m. The morning session consisted of four hours of class concluding by lunchtime, after which lab immediately followed. Lab covered cases on various pathologies to help solidify the material introduced in lecture. We tackled these scenarios in groups of four. The day officially ended around 5:00 p.m., and when it was finally over, we walked home through freezing winds and snow where more studying greeted us. We ate dinner, maybe worked out, watched an episode of *Veep*, slept. The cycle renewed in the morning.

In the beginning of CPP&T, I could be found in the lecture hall each morning, surrounded by my colleagues, coffee in hand. By the end of the first unit, we were dropping like flies. A week after that, just before I finally decided to stop going to class, there were only about thirty others in lecture with me.

It took a year and a half for me to discover, but I had learned that the modern era of medical school involved a lot of self-teaching. Judging by conversations with friends at other medical schools, this was not unique to my experience, and with each passing day, the lack of lecture attendance became an increasingly contentious issue for the administration. The faculty had trouble wrapping their heads around why their students paid so much money in tuition to learn from world-renowned experts only to blow them off when the time came for in-person lectures. Our lecturers were understandably frustrated after investing their limited time into organizing slideshows and three-hour monologues to the just fifteen students in attendance on a good day.

Since most of CPP&T required rote memorization of meticulous details related to hundreds of distinct diseases, most of us had concluded that the name of the game was, more or less, seeing the information enough times to etch it into our brains. Because there was an endless trove of material to get through and only so many hours in a given day, sitting in an academic building for nine hours daily was not an efficient use of time. To accomplish the never-ending list of daily repetitions, I had to find somewhere to trim the fat. For me, lecture slides on the history of lupus and the biology of the pancreatic islet cell were the first to go. With lecture out of the picture, four hours freed up every day. In lieu of attending lecture, on top of tuition and alongside nearly every single one of my colleagues, I paid for subscription services specifically designed to facilitate memorization. In short, we opted to consume the most distilled version of the curriculum, the dehydrated astronaut food version of pathophysiology as opposed to the gourmet five-course meal offered in class, even though we paid for both.

In the depths of Reddit threads dedicated to the preclinical years of medical school, there is a term for these core resources: UFAP. UFAP is not just an amusing acronym, it is a consensus statement for the bare minimum students needed to know in order to succeed on the boards. It stood for UWorld ($500), First Aid ($50), and Pathoma ($85). Curiously, none of these resources were explicitly covered in CPP&T since our course directors had not yet attempted to integrate them into lectures. We only really discovered UFAP through the universal neuroticism which had helped us get into medical school in the first place, connected us with upperclassmen, and encouraged our perusal of online forums like Reddit.

UWorld is the granddaddy of all "question banks." Question

banks vary by company (UWorld, Kaplan, USMLE-Rx, Amboss, etc.) but fundamentally, they share a few overarching characteristics. Each generates more than 2,000 practice questions in the format of the boards (a.k.a. United States Medical Licensing Exam [USMLE] Step 1) with accompanying explanations used to quiz our growing knowledge base. You could sort questions by specific topic or randomize them for general review. Because contemporary research on learning has shown that the most effective means of studying is through self-assessment, I subscribed to two question banks and, between them, tackled anywhere between ten and twenty questions every day, slowly chipping away at the total.

First Aid for the USMLE Step 1 is the medical school bible. This 800-page textbook transcribes every detail, big and small, which students need to know to ace the boards. There is not a single ounce of extraneous information; every line, factoid, and pathology slide pictured in the textbook is testable material. I bought First Aid during MS1 and used it to supplement physiology and microbiology, but by the first day of MS2, I was reading it religiously, attempting to get through each chapter twice before a unit's end.

Lastly, to round out UFAP, Pathoma is an online recorded lecture series narrated by the now famous pathologist, Dr. Hussein Sattar. The resource covers the basics of pathology in detail. The video lectures are accompanied by a 200-page textbook documenting all of the "high-yield," must know facts for the boards. Before a new unit started, I tried to watch these lectures in their entirety at least once.

Because UFAP represents only the tip of the iceberg, many students, myself included, also subscribed to additional applications and websites outside of the curriculum that focused on teaching toward the test. I learned microbiology and pharmacology through cartoons called Sketchy Medical ($600). A subscription to Sketchy offered access to sketches that created memory hooks, much like the Roman Room memory technique. The creators had inventively built rooms integrating each bacterium, virus, and fungus. A single picture included the type of bug (e.g., *Staphylococcus aureus*, *Streptococcus pyogenes*), its armaments (protein A, catalase, urease), disease characteristics (honey-crusted rash, strawberry tongue), patient population (kids, adults, ethnic groups), long-term effects (periprosthetic joint infection, mitral valve disease), and treatment (penicillin, vancomycin). They did the same for each medication and eventually for each disease, too.

Others subscribed to Boards and Beyond ($300) to learn about the mechanisms of biochemistry, neuroanatomy, and pathophysiology. These short clips are structured like Khan Academy videos, teaching specifically to the board exams without any fluff. They dissect hour-long lectures and pare them down into the fifteen-minute SparkNotes version. Over the course of hundreds of lectures, the time savings were enormous.

Most also used an application known as Anki ($0). This includes flashcards which can easily be downloaded onto a computer or phone. Anki gained a large following due to its reliance on the proven principle of "spaced repetition," facilitated by an algorithm that introduces facts at varying intervals in time. Flashcard decks in the Anki Cloud can be uploaded and accessed by any user, and over time, several popular decks began to dominate the scene. These commonly cover facts and even screenshots of pictures presented in First Aid or Pathoma or Sketchy. Disciples of Anki told me that the nearly 10,000 cards in the "Lightyear" or "Zanki" deck would be sufficient to hammer home all the details of Step 1. A user would begin by "unlocking" the appropriate cards from a given unit. A single card presented a question or fill-in-the-blank on one side, and, with the tap of the space bar, the answer would be revealed on the other. Depending on how comfortable a student felt with that particular fact, they could assign a time interval after which it would show up in the future, for example, one day, one week, or one month later. The more times a card was shown, the longer the interval before it showed up again. Like questions in a question bank, the user would unlock a few dozen cards each day and slowly chip away at the total until each card had been adequately mastered.

I tried to love Anki once, but it did not love me back. I thought the facts were delivered in no logical order or context, so it felt like I was memorizing random facts and word associations with no understanding of the bigger picture. Also, because of the way Anki utilizes spaced repetition, it punishes the user for any days taken off. Failure to tackle cards on one day leads them to roll over into the next. Given the pressure imposed on completing all daily assigned cards, many of my classmates lost flexibility in their schedules. At varying points throughout the day, these Anki devotees could be seen hammering away at their space bar in the most frustrating and counterintuitive of settings: in class, during a Super Bowl watch party, in an Uber on the way home, five beers deep after a night out.

Anki represented the extreme of this feeling of perpetually falling behind, but at its core, that was life during second year. There was always more work to be done. Hanging out with friends was a conscious choice to not study and a decision to be paid for later. Every day was a carbon copy of itself, rinsing and repeating the same monotonous daily experience of studying, reviewing, testing. In the midst of this tedium, as quickly as we learned to skip lecture, we lost the brightness in our eyes and the bushiness of our tails.

Class-goer or not, Anki-er or not, we tried to remain motivated because we were told that learning the information was good for patient care. Thankfully, with each new unit, I witnessed the progression toward this goal. No matter a student's chosen study strategy, at some point before test day, a switch would always flip. Like a 1,000-piece puzzle, after all the time spent slogging away trying to fit seemingly similar pieces into a pale blue sky, I would eventually achieve a critical threshold wherein fitting each new fact into a larger picture became easier and easier. Every unit was similar in that way—a slow burn—until everything fell into place all at once. I could see the percent of questions I was getting correct on a given practice test increasing. I volunteered at a free clinic and finally knew something about a patient's chronic kidney disease. At some point, I looked back to realize I had come a long way in just a few months, and that feeling was addicting. It might have been the only thing replenishing the hope that MS2 was trying to beat out of me.

Perhaps more persuasive, though, was the knowledge that the score I would ultimately receive on Step 1 at the end of the year largely determined which field of medicine was available to me—while a good score debatably opened doors, a bad score categorically shut them. With a good score, I could feel comfortable applying into any specialty and potentially any program in the country, but with a bad score, fields like otolaryngology, plastic surgery, neurosurgery, orthopedics, and dermatology would be nothing but pipe dreams. It's remarkable to think one could make it through premed as an undergrad, earn acceptance into medical school, and even succeed in the first two years of medical school but, because of a number from a singular event, could essentially be blacklisted from their aspiration of being a certain type of physician. This was something that students understood but administrators could not comprehend because, when they'd sat for the boards years prior, these barriers did not exist. Step 1 was designed as a licensing exam. At its inception, it was pass-fail, but since it was invariably scored on a numerical system (0–280), residency programs began scrutinizing the number. A higher number meant a more qualified applicant, and over the course of decades, as students studied more and more and scores crept higher and higher, it became a gatekeeper to surgical fields and top-tier residency programs. As generations of medical school deans replaced one another, somewhere in the changing of guards, this evolution was lost on them. To them, the Step 1 score did not determine who would be a good doctor or who would be a bad doctor, and under this framework, it upset them that we paid all this money in tuition to flake on classes and prioritize a score.

Fundamentally, this was what happened. We were skipping classes in pursuit of better test scores, even though we also did not believe Step 1 determined who would be a good or bad doctor. Unfortunately, we did understand that it was, rather, about who would get to be a doctor at all. The scores determined our fates. It was like any currency in that it had the value ascribed to it, and at the time, residency programs valued this more than gold or Bitcoin or a piece of paper called a diploma that said we were MDs. Largely out of this understanding, by the time fresh blooms could be smelled wafting through the air and we had taken our last final of second year, the hard work was only beginning. What followed was a seven-week studying abyss known colloquially as the Dedicated Study Block. "Dedicated" was the time in which no other responsibilities existed other than studying for the boards. It was a protected time in the curriculum for us to burrow away in libraries, put our heads down, and get to work. It concluded the day we took Step I.

Before Dedicated started, I made a schedule of nearly every minute of my life for the next seven weeks. I planned out meals, exercises, wellness lunches, dinners, conferences, everything. A typical weekday during study block started in the library when it opened at 8:00 a.m. If I arrived any later, the whole day would be thrown off. I would warm-up with an overview of a few videos targeting areas of weakness, like antipsychotic drugs, the different lipid controlling medications, or the biochemistry of inborn errors of metabolism. I would then take a forty-question "block" and review it. Each block, similarly to test day, lasted one hour. When this was over, I would review my answers and learn from my mistakes. To get through forty answers, this process averaged another hour and a half. I would aim to take and review two blocks before lunch. Then, I would eat my turkey sandwich while watching more educational videos, and after these twenty minutes had passed, I would take and review another two blocks. Soon enough, it would be 5:00 p.m. and time to go home. Dinner, review my notebook of wrong answers, sleep, do it again the next day.

In my mind, the test was as much about endurance as it was about knowledge base, and to build up this stamina, I took practice tests each Saturday. Each practice test had four blocks in total, so in order to simulate an actual exam environment, I added on three more blocks and a one-hour break to reach eight total hours. When this was over, I charted my progress on an Excel sheet and googled score conversions to get an idea of how

I was performing, which was perpetually below where I had hoped to target. On Sundays, I reviewed my answers. This went on for seven weeks until my official test date.

Because I had taken the MCAT to get into medical school, the test day experience was nothing new. I was used to waking up early and trying to force out a poop at 6:00 a.m. so I wouldn't have that urge in the middle of a question stem. I was used to the downtown Prometric MegaCenter where I would sit for the exam. I was used to getting my fingerprints taken before entering the room, the anxiety before hitting the Start button, the specific snacks I had picked out for my breaks so I wouldn't get too sleepy but also wouldn't be too hungry (fruit leather, Clif Bars, Gatorade). I was also used to the three-week waiting period after the test was over before I eventually got my score, the fatigue and the relief from finally being done with this test for which I'd studied for over two years. Until this point, though, I'm not sure I'd ever been familiar with the feeling of being burnt out.

———

The brain is a gluttonous creature. To support its enormous processing power, it consumes sugar and oxygen faster than any other organ in the body. In the case of an ischemic stroke, a blood clot or traveling cluster of cholesterol lodges itself in a vessel usually narrowed by chronic plaque buildup and prevents the delivery of life-sustaining nutrition to downstream neurons helping with sensation, motor function, blood pressure support, language, or higher-order thinking. Without blood flow, cellular metabolism ceases, and areas of dead and dying tissue begin to form within minutes. Time is brain, we learn, and the faster one can reperfuse the tissue, the better the outcomes. Physicians routinely do this by physically retrieving the clot with endovascular techniques and/or by administering clot-busting medications like tissue plasminogen activator (tPA). If done in a timely manner, they might just salvage the growing circle of dying tissue radiating outward from the tributaries of the artery. This area is called the penumbra, and by definition, it has the potential to be saved.

With all the information, resources, and content, my second year of medical school was one giant penumbra. Each unit, sketch, chapter, audiobook, YouTube video, flash card, and question block was a clot severing ties to what gave me life. It inevitably left me gasping for air. I know it has been said that, in near-death experiences, life flashes before your eyes. People see their most precious memories, their loved ones, what they care about most and cannot live without. I had spent a year metaphorically dying a slow death, ruminating over these questions and considering what it might be that would finally dissolve the clot or who it might be who would come along to scoop it out.

More often than not, I sat in the same dusty cubicle in the Regenstein Library. Under the fluorescent light, I knew my happiness on a given day didn't come from learning about Wegener's granulomatosis with polyangiitis or Paget's disease of the breast. What made me happy was the sound my laptop made when it clicked shut and told me I could leave the library, get on my bike, and pedal home to make salmon curry with a side of zucchini. Every evening, there was always an unmistakable surge of dopamine the minute my teeth were brushed and my head hit the pillow, and in that time between states of existence, with my eyes open and my brain closed, I could finally slow down to welcome the nothingness as it poured over me. I found so much peace in the moments spent fighting off sleep because I knew, if I could have just pressed pause right there in that limbo of darkness, it would have all gone away. The stress would have melted. I would have felt somehow lighter, and the penumbra would have been salvaged. I try not to think too hard about how that which actively made me happy was the very thought of leaving the job that was supposed to bring me joy.

There is a certain vanity carried by those who go into medicine. I remember feeling that way when I was a premed surrounded by business majors, when my friends would wonder out loud about their purpose in life. After graduation, they would be off to fancy jobs in investment banking or venture capital or some other buzzword with which I was vaguely acquainted, and they belabored the point that, deep down, they knew they would be working to make rich people richer, to help big companies consume small companies, to help the opening and closing bell ring out on Wall Street. When five or six or seven o'clock rolled around, they would collect their salaries, and they would ask me if it was okay to feel good about that. I think back to those conversations when, beer in hand, I would do my best to not emanate smugness, knowing that I could always hang my hat on the pretention that, no matter how I felt at that time or how behind I was in studying for a calculus or physics or organic chemistry midterm, I knew I was better than them. These were questions I didn't have to worry about.

In medicine, we get to think we're above other professions. I have participated in numerous workshops on resiliency in healthcare, and this is a theme which is consistently reiterated. We're told, indirectly, that of course a businesswoman or finance executive is going to question their contributions to society because, at the end of the day, they weren't like us. They didn't have this calling. They weren't applying themselves in this specific way to make the world a better place.

Thinking about burnout as an abstract concept, I wonder how it is that I could have ever believed that, because we are healers, we should not experience burnout. I cannot help but consider myopic the idea that morality was what combated disillusionment. By these rules, doctors should feel fully equipped to handle it, if they felt disillusioned at all. The irony of trying to teach this degree of self-importance to trainees is proven year after year by the reported rates of physician burnout (up to 80 percent), suicide (28–40 of every 100,000; twice that of the general population), alcoholism (12.9 percent of males, 21.9 percent of females; more than twice that of the general population), and prescription drug addiction (more than five times that of the general population). These data expose the fallacy shared by so many in medicine: that our jobs define us. What we are not told is that there will come a day when we all learn that there's nothing glamorous about reading the same passage of a textbook three times in a row, tapping away on the spacebar of a computer even on days when we don't want to, spending two minutes charting paperwork to every one spent talking to patients. Someday, we will all realize that it's a rat race, a treadmill, a hamster wheel of never-ending work. For some, it is during the second year of medical school when we ponder what we have to show for it other than a three-digit score; for others, it's years into practice when we look back and ask if we would do it all over again if given the choice.

The whole idea of burnout cannot be summarized as a morality issue. The question that burnout asks at a fundamental level is not what we are going to give to the world at the end of the day nor what is going to be written on our tombstones when we pass—that goes somewhere else in the folder of existential dread. Burnout does ask if we are satisfied with what we are doing, if we fight off sleep because we know that, the minute we slip into unconsciousness, we'll have to wake up and to do it all over again the next day.

There are a lot of aspects of medicine that make me happy. Working with other people gives me energy. I like to learn new things and make people laugh. I find joy in bringing others comfort and being part of a team. To me, this is medicine because it is all I know. But it doesn't have to be. There are hundreds of other jobs out there that satisfy these criteria, and I think I can now better appreciate that, sometimes, these pleasures are not even found strictly within one's job. Self-actualization does not have to be a career thing. Sometimes, it is the simple joys outside of the office: finding the first tulip of the year unfurling as it spirals upward, the smell of the air after it rains, the way droplets of water hang onto tree leaves before falling to the ground, pulled by this force we cannot see but can very much feel. I think it's natural to want more from life. We all want to be happy, to seek fulfillment, to think there is more out there than what we face in the immediate present, to look out the library window and want to be in the sunshine, to think if we could just sprawl out on the grass like a dog for fifteen minutes, then everything would be better.

————

When I was in high school, I went to The Home Depot and procured my very first houseplant. This particular fellow was a feeble-looking Echeveria succulent that I brought home and put in the windowsill above the kitchen sink. It sat there for about two years until I moved out of the house and appointed my mom as its new plant parent. This went smoothly for some time until, one day, her cat ate it. Instead of telling me, she quietly replaced the succulent with a new one. I went on living my life believing this lie, thinking every time I came home that the new, replacement succulent was my original plant child. I didn't find out about the switch until many years after the fact.

Being a kid was so much easier. I was constantly shielded from the world around me. I got to be happy and not bear the burden of responsibility. Sometime after college when I entered the real world, I started to notice my grandparents repeating themselves in conversations over lunch. I was the one leaving a voicemail on my best friend's cell after I learned that his dad had been given six months to live. I got the phone call when a cousin overdosed on opioids. I was on the other end of the table talking to a date about her parents' separation after twenty years and three kids together. I was the one waking up in the middle of the night with a side-splitting pain because my own body decided it was going to start attacking me from the inside out. I am the one wondering if this is the career that I thought I signed up for. I think if it were to happen today, my mom would have told me that her cat ate my succulent.

There is a tendency shared by millennials where we all look around for more. It might not be accurate, but it seems like older generations were happier. For many of them, their paths were laid out in front of them. They went to high school and maybe college, got a job close to home. They married young and had a few kids. They spent the next eighteen or more years of their lives devoted to their children and teens and young adults. Soon enough, they were fifty-year-olds looking toward retirement and grandchildren and hobbies outside of work.

After high school and college, for so many others like me, the next move is not defined. When I graduated from high school, I had no plans of getting hitched or having kids. I felt no ties to my hometown. I didn't owe anybody anything. I was single and unbound by the responsibility of maintaining another's welfare. I made new friends and found a career unlike anything anybody in my family had done before and, in all of this, there was time. There was time to be selfish and stupid. Time to travel and move away from home, time after class or work to watch the game or read or try out a new restaurant, but mostly, there was time to think. After and through all of this thinking, I find myself still in a quarter-life crisis, trying to understand what it is that makes me happy. I turn to social media and see all these perfectly manufactured lives that people put forth for consumption, and I want that for myself. There's a weird sensation that I cannot quite pin down. It's not exactly the feeling of wanting specifically what another person has. I know that isn't it. I don't particularly want to be a homeowner yet or be at that person's rooftop pool or taking care of that new puppy, but I do want what the pictures make them seem like they are feeling, and that is happy.

On New Year's every year when the ball starts to drop and "Auld Lang Syne" plays, the people on TV in Times Square are always kissing. Confetti flies in the background, and I'm usually sitting inside somewhere with a gentle glow on my face, feeling overwhelmingly empty. I don't want to be in Times Square because it's twenty degrees out there, and I know the people dancing onscreen can't feel their fingers or toes. I don't want to be surrounded by strangers, getting stepped on by drunk idiots, or feeling the urgent need to urinate but not wanting to give up the spot I'd elbowed my way into. I don't want to be them, though I do feel something toward them. I wish there were a word in the English language that could capture that dissatisfaction of half-baked jealousy so that I could at least understand it better. A nostalgia, a yearning for something that one has never experienced.

As I neared the end of MS2, from a cubicle in the library looking out the window, I could not help but wonder which side of the glass I wanted to be on. And at least at that time, I was on the inside.[i]

---

[i]   In response to growing criticism about the overemphasis of a single metric, in 2022, the USMLE services transitioned to a pass-fail format for Step 1. The shift was intended to promote a more holistic approach to medical education. Step 2 and Step 3 remain on a three-digit score reporting system.

7

THRESHOLDS

Life is often compared to a marathon, but I think it is more like being a sprinter; long stretches of hard work punctuated by brief moments in which we are given the opportunity to perform at our best.

—Michael Johnson

MEDICAL SCHOOL, in many ways, is a lot like high school. We either walked to school each day or took the bus. We were all given lockers to store our backpacks and textbooks, and we hung out at them in between classes. There were clubs and intramural sports we had the option of joining in our free time, too. By the end of the second year, friend groups were firmly established, and we got dressed up together each spring to go to our version of prom. Everybody knew everybody, and nothing stayed a secret for very long. Whether they were true or not, rumors spread quickly.

"Did you know that Jason is secretly interested in dating Gena?"

"So, Ryan's Jamie is actually a man?"

"Did somebody say throuple?!?"

What distinguished medical school from high school, besides the workload and cadavers, was that, instead of there being cool kids or jocks or goths, we were all united, deep down, by this universal truth that we were nerds. And there was nothing quite like facing the biggest examination of our lives to reinforce this fact.

Studying for Step 1 was inherently different than for the Scholastic Assessment Test (SAT) or the MCAT. Unlike those examinations, Step 1 could only be taken once; there were no do-overs. Whatever score we obtained would be on our residency applications, and, again, the question was never whether we would pass the boards but rather how high (or low) the number would be, because it ultimately would determine which specialty a residency applicant might be competitive in. This, very likely, was the first time in our lives we'd faced a definitive checkpoint.

Because of this, the Step 1 score release day carried an unprecedented level of stress. Unfortunately, there also was a painstakingly long three-week delay after the exam; this was when the curve was set. During this time, I slowly relearned what it meant to be a human. The vitamin D levels in my body began to normalize as I emerged from my library cocoon and rediscovered my hobbies. Afternoons spent waiting included bike rides five miles down the lakeshore and carrying a Callaway Prototype 6 iron in a tiny string bag to a beat-up driving range, where I could slice golf balls into the weeds and sip on India pale ales with my classmates, John and Bobby. In between range sessions, we would pontificate on how unfair it was to put so much emphasis on a test score, and how there was inherent value to doctors in specialties that did not enforce this standard so stringently.

When the day of my score release came around, I felt sick to my stomach. I had played mental gymnastics for the previous two years, hedging my bets, trying to convince myself that I might be satisfied going into any specialty. Deep down, though, I knew that I wanted to enter a specialty that required a high boards score. I had put everything I had into the first two years of medical school, and I'd sacrificed two months of my life to a dedicated study period, hoping it would be enough.

I tried to approach the score release practically. I picked a number below which I would allow myself to be upset. I picked a score range in the right half of the bell curve that would satisfy a threshold any residency program might theoretically set as a screening tool, and if I fell within this range, I told myself to feel happy because my dreams would still be possible. I also allowed my imagination to wander, and I picked a number above which I would know that I had met my goal, in which case I would feel ecstatic knowing that I would be more qualified than most medical students when the next application season came around.

The e-mail came through when I was at home. I calmly gathered my belongings and walked into my bedroom before taking a deep breath, saying a quick prayer, then clicking on the link. When the website finally refreshed, I learned that I had fallen into the second bucket, the range that kept my dreams alive. I hadn't quite met my goal, but then again, I refused to beat myself up because I had accomplished something substantial. I felt that my hard work was reflected in the score, and a weight had not just been lifted but had been ejected off my back. I closed out the 20 tabs that were open on my Google Chrome browser, and I texted the score to the family group chat.

When I walked out of my room, I saw Ryan smiling at his phone.

"How did things go?" he asked.

With a sigh of relief, I finally said out loud, "I'm interested in orthopedic surgery."

MS3

8

THE WARDS

He sought his former accustomed fear of death and did not find it. 'Where is it? What death?' There was no fear because there was no death. In place of death there was light.

—Leo Tolstoy, *The Death of Ivan Ilych*

THE SOLE PURPOSE of the first two years of medical school was creating a foundation that would serve us well when we were off on our clinical rotations. On the spectrum of human interaction, those first two years swung more toward the side of being an introvert's paradise. Most days were spent with our faces buried in our laptops, tucked away in the corner of a library, attempting to master information found in a textbook. It did not test inter-personal skills nor humanism nor the art of medicine itself.

With the passing of part one of the boards, we transitioned out of the preclinical years and onto the wards. In this setting, we accepted increased responsibility, which we looked toward with great expectation. We were now upperclassmen, and we would be expected to care for our patients, to advocate for them, to put forth treatment plans which would eventually get them home to their loved ones. We would be trusted to write progress notes in the electronic medical record; call families, consultants, and staff with updates; and perform rudimentary procedures under the supervision of more experienced physicians. We would conduct our own physical exams, make opening incisions, and get "pimped" into the earth by our seniors (i.e., grilled with a series of questions about a patient's case or medical topic, a hazing ritual/pastime of medicine aimed at assessing a trainee's knowledge, critical thinking skills, and ability to apply medical knowledge to clinical situations). In that way, it was very exciting. This was what we came to medical school to do.

My school offered seven core MS3 rotations in total. Each ranged anywhere from four to twelve weeks in duration. The rotations included what we called the "triplet" (family medicine, psychiatry, neurology), the "doublet" (obstetrics and gynecology, pediatrics), general surgery, and general internal medicine. Depending on the length of the rotation, we also had our pick of several two-week elective blocks to explore other disciplines like emergency medicine, cardiology, and a variety of surgical subspecialties.

The day-to-day schedule ranged from the 4:30 a.m. wake up times on surgery to strolling into the psych wards at 9:00 a.m. On arrival, we would chat with the bedside nurse and look up overnight events for the two to four patients under our care. Later that morning, we would present these patients to the care team on rounds. We would then log into the medical record and document events that took place over the past 24 hours, as well as the day's plan. We spent most afternoons in scheduled lectures, in impromptu chalk talks delivered by the residents or waiting for something interesting to happen (echocardiogram, chest tube placement, cases in the operating room). The days would end when a benevolent resident noticed that we still existed and would dismiss us to go home. On the more laid-back rotations, this could happen as early as 2:00 or 3:00 p.m. But if the residents were swamped, in a bad mood, or stuck in a complicated surgical case, this could be as late as nine or ten o'clock at night, if not later. Once home, we would whip up a quick meal and study for the upcoming "shelf exam," a national standardized test taken at the end of each clerkship and factoring into our overall grade for the rotation.

In all of the rotations, the hierarchy is largely consistent. The medical student works directly with a first-year resident, also referred to as an intern. The first-year resident, in turn, reports to a more senior resident with somewhere between two to six more years of experience. Lastly, the senior resident reports to an attending physician. As the boss, the "attending" must approve all plans. He or she signs off on all orders and "lays eyes" on each patient daily.

In total, I spent 365 days on the wards as a third-year medical student, and during this time, a lot of things happened. Most of them were not necessarily happening to me, but they certainly were happening around me. The hospital is a crazy place, filled with dying patients and the buzzing people—nurses, trainees, and full-blown doctors—trying to keep them alive. Sprinkled into this pandemonium is a slurry of new social norms and personalities and the constant performative nature of "objective" evaluations in this setting. From the stress of learning the fundamentals of each medical specialty to everything involved in caring for another person, the third year was abundantly more stressful than the second year, but it was also more fun. Most days were filled with firsts:

- First code
- First overnight shift
- First diagnosis cinched
- First skin laceration repaired
- First time retracting in surgery
- First time getting locked in the stairwell while pre-rounding
- First time accidentally following a resident into the bathroom
- First time forgetting to leave a callback number on a consult page
- First time stealing saltines from the hospital's nourishment rooms
- First time having pants fall down in the OR
- First time saying to an attending, "I don't think I have the vocabulary to answer the question you just asked me."
- First time frantically searching for a staple remover in the supply closet while the team waited by the patient's room on rounds

As the year wound to an end and I became more aware of the deadline to decide on a specialty, I understood that many of my firsts would also be lasts:

- (Hopefully) last time accidentally chugging cold brew

concentrate before a surgery and having to leave the
OR because of explosive diarrhea

- Last time emailing the entire school listserv about
the status of my nipples to promote a wellness event
- Last time pretending to be busy while the intern
stared at his computer
- Last time carrying fifteen extra pens in the pockets of
my white coat
- Last time reporting the news that the margins were
clear
- Last full-length psychiatric history
- Last well-child checkup
- Last baby delivered

I look back on many of these moments with fond remembrance, but I also know that, amid these firsts and lasts, the most rewarding part of the third year had nothing to do with the process of applying knowledge. What made it so remarkable were the highs and lows of salvation and suffering, the individual stories of triumph and heartbreak that I witnessed every day and, at times, had the privilege of playing a small role in. The lessons I took with me out of the third year stemmed mostly from the understanding that the people I met on the wards weren't heart failure patients or trauma victims or cases of appendicitis. Rather, they were people first—people who just happened to be patients at the point in time when their lives intersected with mine. In the first framing, the disease describes a person; in the other, it is but a qualifier denoting the condition afflicting an individual life.

Every day, I wrote notes about patients in their charts. They were supposed to be impersonal accounts of symptoms and data. I would start with a descriptor of the problem and the chief complaint:

> *Mr. X is a 55-year-old male presenting with chest pain*
> *for two hours in duration.*

I would go on to describe the pain in detail along with any associated symptoms and prior medical and surgical history. I included relevant tobacco or drug use, family history, labs, imaging (if any), and conclude with an assessment:

> *History and physical consistent with gastroesophageal*
> *reflux disease (GERD). Differential includes*
> *cardiac (myocardial infarction, angina),*
> *pulmonary (pneumothorax, pulmonary embolism,*
> *pneumonia), and musculoskeletal (trauma, costo-*
> *chondritis) though low concern at this time. Will*
> *start on a proton pump inhibitor. Return precau-*
> *tions discussed.*

It would have been frivolous to say that he will have been married to his wife for twenty years this upcoming Friday or to include how he volunteers at the YMCA in his free time. The record does not care that he still uses a flip phone or that his daughter thinks he is the most eloquent man she has ever met, though these details might just be what my patients wanted me to know the most. It is so interesting how narratives shape us.

Over the course of the year, there were countless faces that made their way out of my memory. Each one's experience in the hospital relegated to a medical record number, troponin and calcium levels, CT scans and chest X-rays. I feel some degree of regret looking out at this sea of hundreds, faces with no defining characteristics attached to bodies with amorphous figures, crying out in voices with generic pitches. For many of these characters, no matter how hard I try, the synapses in the fusiform gyrus of my temporal lobe no longer exist, and I cannot recognize that which I should. Reverse déjà vu, a jamais vu of sorts.

For a select few, their memories forge on. The harsh odor of stomach acid suctioned from a nasogastric tube will always take me back to a specific room in the Center for Care and Discovery where, most days, I could see an open abdomen healing by secondary intention. The amber color of bowel sweat pooling in an ileostomy bag will forever be linked to a greying beard and a balding head. Some of these faces haunt me, while others I remember with reverence, but all of them I will carry with me throughout my career, for their attitudes and insight and circumstances have taught me more than medicine ever could. In one way or another, they have managed to shape their own narratives. These are the stories that I would like to share.

9

RAHEEM

Only that day dawns to which we are awake. There is more day to dawn. The sun is but a morning star.

—Henry David Thoreau, *Walden*

IN BIOLOGY, we learn that form follows function, and in the case of hemoglobin, this rule reigns supreme. Hemoglobin is the main component of a red blood cell, which is inherently designed to carry oxygen. This is its purpose in life; a screw screws, a hammer hammers, a red blood cell carries oxygen.

To this end, hemoglobin is a beautifully complex system. The largest of its parts are four subunits, two alphas and two betas. In healthy adults, two dimers are formed from one alpha and one beta.

Each hemoglobin subunit is home to an atom of iron (Fe^{2+}), its positive charge constantly seeking a negatively charged mate, perhaps better known as oxygen (O^{2-}). The two alpha-beta dimers are important in that their asymmetry allows for minor changes in shape. The binding of one oxygen to one iron atom in one subunit induces the slightest of changes to the shape of the whole molecule such that other oxygen atoms are also more likely to bind to the other subunits. In other words, once one oxygen is bound, the affinity for oxygen is now higher for subunit number two. Once two oxygen atoms are bound, the affinity for oxygen is higher for subunit number three. And it's even higher for subunit number four, such that the probability of hemoglobin being completely saturated with oxygen increases in a sigmoid fashion as more oxygen atoms are recruited. This is most likely to occur in high-oxygen environments like the lungs.

The converse is also true. Once one oxygen falls off, the affinity decreases rapidly. Therefore, the odds that other oxygen atoms also fall off increase as well. This occurs in low-oxygen environments like the capillaries of the kidneys, liver, and spleen, which require oxygen to sustain metabolism and ultimately life. Because of the important role that hemoglobin plays, in most hospitalized patients, it is measured daily. Its level informs providers of occult sources of blood loss, such as a bleeding surgical incision.

A normal hemoglobin concentration ranges from 12–17 grams per deciliter (g/dL). It's not a static number, and it fluctuates by as much as 0.2 g/dL per day. Variability depends on factors like hydration (which changes overall blood volume), blood loss (from a wound or menstruation), or minor lab error. Doctors carefully monitor abnormally low hemoglobin levels, given research studies consistently demonstrate that levels below 7.0 g/dL can increase the risk for adverse outcomes like heart attacks, heart failure, infection, and death. Because of this threat, if a patient has a hemoglobin reading below that threshold, they are typically given blood. The lowest I had seen earlier in my third year was around 4.8 g/dL. That patient was experiencing dizziness to the point of losing consciousness when standing, heart palpitations, and shortness of breath. She was transfused with three units of blood in the ED.

Raheem Clark[i] arrived at the hospital with a hemoglobin level of 2.0 g/dL. He was "found down" in the street on a summer afternoon and was admitted to the intensive care unit clinging to life. There, he was immediately transfused until his vital signs stabilized. After a few days, I met him when he was transferred to my service, internal medicine.

Mr. Clark was cachectic. This is not a kind descriptor, but it is accurate and illustrative. The word cachectic literally means "wasting," and it is usually reserved to describe the appearance of those who have undergone a severe, prolonged assault on the body like what we see with acquired immunodeficiency syndrome (AIDS), chronic kidney disease, or leukemia. In this case, I saw it in his eyes, which sat deeply within their sockets, the fat pads of days prior long since tarnished. I saw it in his maxilla, casting dark shadows over his sunken cheeks, covered, futilely, by the patches of his curly, black beard. I saw it in the ribs I could count when listening to his heart thump, thump, thumping away at irregular intervals. In his slender fingers, jutting out like gnarled roots, marred at the joints by lopsided, stonelike deposits characteristic of gouty tophi.

---

[i] All patient examples are based on real clinical cases; however, names, identifying details, and certain circumstances have been altered to protect patient privacy.

As extreme as the presentation was, all of us were considering the same differential. When an older gentleman is admitted with chronic blood loss, the most likely source is gastrointestinal in origin. The ranges of diagnoses included a bleeding stomach or small intestinal (duodenal) ulcer, esophageal varices, or conceivably more likely, colon cancer.

The workup for all these maladies was also rather straightforward. We'd first need an esophagogastroduodenoscopy, or EGD for short. This entails a small camera, or scope, being inserted through the mouth, down the esophagus, and into the duodenum to visualize the upper part of the gastrointestinal (GI) tract. Even if we found a bleed with this test, however, to rule out the "must-not-miss" diagnosis of cancer and the possibility of two separate sources of bleeding (i.e., one upper GI and one lower), we'd need to visualize the lower half of the GI tract. This is accomplished with a colonoscopy.

After meeting Mr. Clark, I laid out my plan: "Sir, I am afraid that you may be bleeding along your gastrointestinal tract. We would like to look with a few tests to confirm before we are able to start treatment. One test requires a camera to be inserted through your mouth; this is called an EGD. The other requires a camera in your rectum, also known as a colonoscopy. Both are relatively short procedures, and you would be provided medications throughout to make you as comfortable as possible."

Mr. Clark was as hard to read as he was reticent, and to my surprise, he refused. His eyes averted my gaze; he did not offer fear nor anger, but he remained steadfast in his defiance. In the face of such a challenge, I fell back on my training. After all, I had seen this before and could hear the voices of my professors lecturing: "meet the patient where they are at," "share the decision-making," "empathize with their situation."

I tried, "Can you tell me a little more about your concerns with the test?"

"I don't know. I don't want it."

I tried again, "What do you like to do outside of the hospital? We can try to get you back to that. I think this is the best way we can help you."

"Yes, but I don't want anything up there."

And again, gently, "I am worried there is a cancer potentially growing in your colon. If we can identify it, we can treat it."

"No, thank you."

And again, more firmly this time, "If we can't localize the source of your bleeding, you could die."

"I don't want anything in my bottom."

"But Mr. Clark, you have a fecal management system in your rectum right now. Don't you want us to get that out?"

"I just don't want anything up there ..."

With each conversation, I could feel his position becoming more and more entrenched. I was losing him. My attending did not have any better luck. On Mr. Clark's fourth hospital day, after lunch, I received a page from his nurse: "GI bleed." I arrived in his room with my senior resident to find half a liter of bright red blood in his fecal management system. Soon after, he consented to two units of blood. When asked about the possibility of getting the colonoscopy, he again refused.

———

A few months later, when I was on the residency interview trail, a surgeon asked me about my favorite class in medical school. As somebody applying into a surgical subspecialty, my knee-jerk reaction was anatomy. Learning about the muscles of the body and the way they exert forces on bones to mobilize joints fascinated me. Visualizing the snaking courses of vasculature, how red arteries and blue veins twisted around precious white nerves, was awe-inspiring. But my answer, after working for nearly a year on various care teams in different settings, was medical ethics.

Ethics is not innately objective; it is humanistic. And for me, it was also the class that most closely mirrored the clinical year. Medicine, for all its facts and figures, is not black and white. Each day, we face the in-between. To operate or not operate. To push a medication or hold off on treatment. To hospitalize or send home. The grey is what makes medicine a form of art. In the grey of tough decisions, we are taught that we must respect the four main pillars of medical ethics: autonomy, beneficence (do good), non-maleficence (do no harm), and justice.

I helped care for a patient on my psychiatry rotation who was admitted with a relatively rare condition called postpartum psychosis (incidence of about one in 1000 live births). It usually involves the mother losing touch with reality and, often, attempting self-harm or harm of her newborn. For these reasons, mothers with postpartum psychosis are involuntarily hospitalized and separated from their child until they can receive the appropriate treatment. Treatment in this case involves antipsychotic medications usually administered via intramuscular injection.

The history I was signed out when I walked into the hospital that morning was that this patient was brought in by her husband in a state of disarray. The prior evening, she had taken the lipstick out of her purse and started drawing pictures on the windows and mirrors. Additionally, she was rearranging furniture and reportedly calling her baby by her dog's name. During my interview with her, I learned a few more details. The patient told me that, for the past few days, her husband had fallen ill. Because of this, all the baby duties had shifted to her. As a result, she was running on only a few hours of sleep while caring for her child, breastfeeding, cooking, and cleaning. She admitted to me that she was stressed. Her husband must have noticed and offered her a hit of marijuana. The next part of the story is, more or less, information collected from collateral and consistent with the story I heard on arrival. It included lipstick, windows, and a drive to the ED in the middle of the night. By the time I had interviewed her, her acute episode had resolved. Nevertheless, out of an abundance of caution, my supervisor ended up keeping her hospitalized. The official diagnosis was postpartum psychosis.

This patient's stay lasted four days in total. It was likely more protracted because she did not want to take antipsychotic medications, believing 1) that she was not in a state of psychosis and 2) that the medication, once in her bloodstream, could get in her breast milk and affect her baby. Both of these were reasonable concerns. During her hospitalization, she yelled, she cried, and she threatened litigation. Her feelings are perhaps best summarized by paraphrasing some of her own words:

"Do you want to know why I seem manic right now? It's because my husband is incompetent. He hasn't been taking care of our kid because he's sick, so I've been doing everything. I was brought to the ED against my will, I am stuck here in the psych ward against my will, and I had my baby taken away from me against my will. So, you want to know why I am upset? I am humiliated, I am indignant, I am *fucking* pissed, and I will sue you into the ground for taking my child away from me."

Her speech gave me chills. Would I not do the exact same

thing for my baby? What if I were the attending? Could I live
with myself, separating a mother from her child, not even letting
her leave the room to breastfeed? But what if the attending, in
all his years of experience, was right, and she ended up truly
being psychotic and, upon discharge, promptly harmed herself
or murdered her baby? Was involuntary hospitalization and
separation of mother and child in itself a beneficent action?

———

On my general surgery rotation, I took care of a man who
received a neobladder. In a neobladder procedure, the original
bladder is removed because it is no longer viable (due to
cancer in this case). A new bladder is then created using the
small intestine. A large segment is removed and the two
endpieces are stitched together to reconnect the bowels, while
the middle portion is opened and fastened into an overlapping
pouch capable of holding urine. The ureters coming from the
kidneys are then attached to the top of the neobladder, and the
urethra is anastomosed to the bottom. All of this is made
possible because the intestinal cells lining the neobladder, over
a series of weeks and only after being exposed to urine for a
prolonged duration, transform from intestinal cells into
urothelial cells, the same kind found in the patient's original
bladder.

This procedure really is a testament to the resiliency and
adaptability of the human body. It's also experimental and
highly risky. The intern with whom I was working prior to the
procedure start, who was in fact training to be a urologist, said to
me, "This is really cool, but if I were the patient, I personally
wouldn't elect this procedure. I get that he wants to maintain a

sense of control, but I'd take a urine bag any day," a reference to the patient's alternative, a urostomy.

This patient's surgery was a success in the sense that the neobladder was created, but soon, an abnormal connection, or fistula tract, formed between the neobladder and his abdominal wall. With urine freely draining to the outside world, his incision became infected. He was then sent back to the OR to irrigate, debride, and pack the wound. He had a midline incision the size of a football draining for weeks. He had a tube inserted into his nose for most of his hospital stay to protect his sutured small bowel, which now was having trouble propelling gastric contents forward. His mouth was in a state of permanent aridity. He stank of stomach acid. Urine slowly dribbled onto his abdomen until the fistula closed. He stayed in the hospital for nearly a month, and once home, his quality of life looked bleak.

First, do no harm. How much harm had we caused in trying to help?

———

In neurology, my goal by the end of the rotation was to learn how to perform a lumbar puncture. To me, that represented the main procedural skill on the rotation. The rest was more medicine oriented: performing a proficient neurological exam, localizing strokes, and documenting consistent and accurate examination findings. But the lumbar puncture excited me. It involved taking a long, hollow needle and boring through the midline back right over the spine. From the practice sessions on training dummies, I knew I had to insert the needle at an upward trajectory, mirroring the angle formed by the vertebral spines and threading though the narrow opening. Once in, I would feel a pop as I poked through the ligamentum flavum and into the dura mater, a protective sheath surrounding, at that level, the cauda equina (a collection of nerves at the terminal end of the spinal cord). When I was inside, I could then harvest the cerebrospinal fluid bathing the brain and spinal cord.

This procedure is important for a number of reasons. In some patients with meningitis, it can reveal infection. For select others, the cerebrospinal fluid we collect can be analyzed to detect inflammatory neurological conditions like Guillain-Barré syndrome or multiple sclerosis. For others still, we can drain some cerebrospinal fluid to relieve headaches and nausea caused by the pressure within the central nervous system simply being too high, as in the case of pseudotumor cerebri.

In neurology clinic, I worked with one other co-student. We would see patients with the residents, and they would teach us when things slowed down. When we arrived at clinic, to my delight, we were informed that two afternoon patients needed spinal taps. My co-student knew that I was excited about this procedure and graciously offered to let me take the first "stab" at it.

My patient was a large woman who arrived on a bus that serviced the surrounding lower-income neighborhoods on the south side of Chicago. She was, in fact, suffering from pseudo-tumor cerebri. Because of her medical condition, this was not her first lumbar puncture and certainly would not be her last, but I was very thankful for her generosity in granting me permission to try a spinal tap, and for the residents allowing me to give it a shot.

The procedure went slowly but without hiccups. My resident and the attending physician stood behind, guiding me through the procedure, offering tips when I ran into the L3 vertebra and staying quiet when I needed to focus. After a few minutes, I saw that sweet champagne-colored fluid telling me I was in. It was amazing.

The second patient was assigned to my co-student. After watching my success, he was undoubtedly eager for his shot. Before we stepped into her room, however, we both heard murmurs outside coming from the resident workroom.

"Gold bar. She's a gold bar patient."

At the hospital where I trained, we used a secure electronic medical record for patient charts. When you clicked on a patient, a host of demographic information displayed across the top. Age, sex, allergies, medications, prior diagnoses, primary care provider. This was all broadcast on a pale blue, rectangular backdrop. For this particular patient, the above information was plastered in gold. Apparently, this meant the patient was a major donor to the hospital. Because of this designation, the attending physician saw her immediately after she was roomed. From the hallway, my classmate and I peered in, catching a glimpse of her diamond-studded ears and her husband's designer suit as the door swung shut. After some time, the attending emerged from the lumbar puncture victorious and sent them on their way.

The way the same, standard procedure played out for two patients could not have been much more different. For the first patient, a nervous medical student was given the space to learn. For the second, only the practiced hands of an attending—not even a resident—were deemed worthy of this responsibility. Is this just?

———

On day six of Mr. Clark's hospital stay, two days after the first GI bleed, he bled again. Once more, he accepted the blood and refused the colonoscopy. That day, we paged palliative care. With Mr. Clark, no amount of my recommending, explaining, questioning, or pleading could get him to change his mind. I pushed so hard because I knew that, if we could find the source, we could stop his bleeding. We could resect the tumor. We could potentially prolong his life by years. Also, to the best of my judgement, and in conversations outside of this specific topic, all signs pointed to his wanting to get better, especially since he was accepting other life-sustaining treatments in the form of blood transfusions, nutritional supplementation, and fluids. For all my trying, the harder I pushed, the more he pushed back, and I knew at a certain point, I had to stop and respect his autonomy. If he knew the risks and the benefits, and if he was of sound mind and had decision-making capacity, then he had the right to provide, and to refuse, consent.

Under my care, I watched as his cachexia failed to improve; I received the page for the rapid response when he suffered a third GI bleed; I was there for his final transfusion, bumping him up, for the time being, to a stable hemoglobin of 8.6 g/dL; and I was there when he told me "no" for the last time and was discharged back to the community, where I am sure he passed away.

10

BABY A AND BABY B

We're in the business of inspiration, Joe, but it isn't often we find ourselves inspired.

—Disney and Pixar's *Soul*

IN ANY PREGNANCY, the health of the unborn fetus is frequently assessed using an abdominal ultrasound. This imaging modality offers real-time pictures of the fetus' position inside the uterus, its crown-rump length, head size, heart, reproductive organs, and so on.

In twin pregnancies, because there is more than one individual present, each is given a name. The baby visualized on the ultrasound closest to the birth canal becomes Baby A, and the other, further away, is labeled Baby B. When I heard this in the orientation to my obstetrics and gynecology clerkship, I was admittedly feeling pretty zealous. There might not have been a single thing in medical school that I looked toward with such anticipation as delivering a baby. Ushering life into the world with my bare hands, what could be cooler than that? The following cases were not twin gestations in the sense that the babies came from the same womb, but they did represent my first two experiences participating in the delivery of another human life, mere hours apart.

Baby A was a vaginal birth. I met her mom when her cervix was about three centimeters dilated. In the language of obstetrics, this was nothing concerning. A normal, nonpregnant cervix remains "closed" at zero centimeters. In the hours leading up to the delivery of a newborn, as the uterus begins to contract more and more frequently, a series of hormones induce chemical changes to the shape and texture of the cervix. In time, it softens, effaces, and slowly begins to dilate such that a baby's head can traverse the birth canal, through the vagina, and out into the expectant hands of a caretaker. From zero to about six centimeters in diameter, the process of cervical dilation occurs slowly over the course of many hours, and in some cases, even days. When the cervix finally gets to six centimeters, however, the timer starts ticking. At this inflection point, a typical cervix will begin dilating at a standard rate of roughly 1.2–1.5 centimeters per hour until it achieves a final diameter of ten centimeters. Once there, the pushing commences.

Sometimes, though, this process can become too protracted, and if the rate of change slows or even stops, mom has bought herself extra attention because failure of progression can cause both fetal and maternal stress, including umbilical cord compression, fatigue, and what providers fear, late decelerations. There are a number of different types of decelerations, but "late decels" means the placenta, in some manner or another, has been compromised. A baby with late decels needs to get out.

––––––

Baby B was a *planned* vaginal birth. She was rushed into the operating room with late decelerations due to arrest of labor. I met her mom on the way to the preoperative holding area prior to her emergent cesarean section. She was scared and so was I. This would be my first time scrubbing into an OR.

The process of scrubbing in has become a highly regimented ordeal. Its importance cannot be overstated, as failure to maintain sterile technique can introduce unwelcome microbes into an open cavity and result in serious infection and other patient morbidity (and potentially mortality). Throughout the entirety of the procedure as well, maintaining a sterile field remains at the forefront of patient safety priorities. Later in the rotation, I would come face to face with the veracity with which some surgeons emphasize sterility.

I spent one afternoon working with the gynecologic oncology service. Our agenda for the day involved removing a patient's uterus and cervix to treat recently discovered uterine cancer. This surgery utilized laparoscopy, or small port sites on the abdomen through which instruments were inserted. To fully excise the uterus and manipulate its position within the abdominal cavity, a joystick-like apparatus was usually inserted through the vagina. The far end of the joystick was faceted with a wide, flat brim that rested against the cervix when fully in place. From the outside, the uterus could be "driven" with the blunt, near end to improve the visibility and precision of each cut inside the abdomen. Much like the way an airplane is flown, pulling back on the knob cranked the uterus anterior (up toward the belly button), and pushing the knob away moved the uterus posterior (back toward the spine). Likewise, from the angle of the driver between the patient's legs, rotating counterclockwise moved the uterus to the left, and clockwise moved it to the right. The feedback from each joystick movement was relayed via a camera port to a small TV screen from the vantage point of the resident aiming the camera, usually from the top down (from the head pointing toward the feet).

Maneuvering the uterus in this way was somewhat counter-intuitive, requiring a keen understanding of spatial orientation since the vantage point of the uterus driver was opposite that of the surgeon. This was my job for the procedure, and I found myself sitting on a stool in between the patient's legs for five hours that day. As we neared the finish line, making our final cuts on the vaginal cuff, my job became even more critical. When I thought the uterus needed to be anteverted, I cranked back on the stick. When it needed to go to the patient's left, I rotated clockwise and angled my hands to the left, pushing with all my might back to the right.

Still, despite my efforts, my attending was not satisfied with the visibility that these maneuvers offered, and after my several failed attempts to adjust to his constructive criticism, he sought to correct the issue himself. From my perch, out of the corner of my eye, I caught a glimmer of latex reaching around the patient's leg and quickly closing in on the joystick. Unfortu-nately, my head was situated between the patient's leg and the joystick, and despite my reflexive lurch backward, my face caught the blow of the surgeon's open hand. In his attempt to manipulate the uterus himself, the surgeon dealt me a swift, inadvertent slap. To my bewilderment, he responded, "Oh, my hand is contaminated!" before leaving the procedure to rescrub. I stood up, quietly excused myself, and left the OR to clean myself up.

On the day of Baby B's anticipated debut, none of this had happened yet—I had never donned a pale blue surgical gown, but I needed to scrub in. As I had learned in training sessions, the process was to last no less than two and half minutes. It involved a sponge, a special antibacterial soap, and a systematic washing from fingertip to elbow, including attention first to the nail beds, then the four planes of each individual finger, the back of the hand followed by the palms, and finally, the fore-arms. Once finished, I would need to rinse off, being careful not to touch the sink in the process, the doorknob on my way into the room, or anything from there on out that was not sterile in itself. The day prior, I had swallowed my pride and asked a resident to give me a rudimentary tour of the OR. She'd told me, "Here is the sink where you'll scrub in. Here are the gowns. Here are the gloves. Try to scrub early so you can help with setup."

Because of the emergent nature of the procedure, by the time I had arrived in the OR, the patient was already on the operating table being prepped with a betadine sponge-stick for an imminent start. I left to perform my hand washing, and once finished, I backed into the room, making an earnest effort not to touch the handle as I reentered, realizing only then that, some-how, everybody else had already managed to scrub, gown, and glove, and they were now all waiting on me to finish. I looked like a baby deer caught in the headlights, holding my lanky arms high in the air, beads of water dripping down onto my shoes. The scrub tech fired off a cheap shot, "You need to scrub faster," before physically placing my now gowned and gloved hands onto the sterile field in the patient's lap.

Baby A had progressed as expected. Her mother's contractions were now occurring every two minutes, down from five, and while she'd refused an epidural earlier in the day, she was now requesting another means of pain control. Because it was too late for an epidural, in return, she was offered a medication known as Dilaudid in its place, a frequently used opioid analgesic. The next hour passed quickly and less painfully, and soon enough, she arrived at ten centimeters. I put on boots and shimmied into my oversized gown to cover my baggy scrubs. A natural birth is not a sterile procedure, but we don personal protective equipment nonetheless, more so for our own defense —to keep blood, feces, and other fluid off our clothes.

"One, two, three ... ten."

"PUSH PUSH PUSH PUSH PUSH ... You're doing great. Okay, now rest for a minute."

Mom's legs were being held on one side by her husband, on another by a nurse. I found my spot between her legs, ready for the most important catch of my life. While we waited for another contraction to set off a new round of pushing, I ran through my game plan.

Videos had shown me what to expect, and in my shadowing experiences the past few days, I had witnessed this part play out from the back of the room. The baby's head would begin to crown, and as it descended, the doctor delivering the baby would be expected to protect the perineum, applying downward pressure below the vaginal opening with their dominant hand to minimize the degree of tearing. As the baby's head surfaced, it would be important to rotate the body into the correct position to facilitate delivery of the front, then back shoulder past the narrowing of the ischial spines and pubic symphysis. Once the shoulders cleared, it was smooth sailing: legs, then placenta, then stiches if needed. With the baby out, we would suction amniotic fluid from its mouth with a small plunger to help it breathe, dry it off with a towel to preserve its warmth, and finally place it atop mom's chest for precious skin-to-skin contact.

This time, it was my turn. It would be my hands protecting the perineum, my hands rotating the head, cushioning its descent, gripping with all my might so as not to drop this slippery manifestation of life, of love. To bring into the world a being full of future happiness, heartbreak, hope, and healing. Full of potential for good and for change. She had no idea what she signed up for, the genesis of a tragicomedy in which I was but a peripheral character.

––––––––

In Baby B's operating room, mom chatted quietly with her husband, who sat next to her at the head of the table, the two of them shielded from our temporary office by a makeshift wall in the form of a large blue drape. I found it remarkable that mom would be awake the entire time during the C-section, anesthetized not by the usual cocktail of systemic drugs but instead from the waist down by a spinal block. It wasn't always this way, I later discovered, but you can imagine why this method was preferred. In another life, mom would go into the operating room pregnant, fully conscious. She would be put to sleep for surgery and, during this time, her baby would be safely and efficiently delivered via C-section. Later, mom would wake up from surgery, look down, and be forced to infer that this new baby on her chest was hers. Consciousness during one's childbirth turned out to be such a crucial factor to a mother's perceived closeness and emotional connection to her newborn that now, when possible, moms remain awake. When a spinal block is employed, patients do not feel pain, but they can experience the pressure of the delivery, hear the first cry of their newborn, and be physically and mentally present for the culmination of a nine-month journey.

From my position during the procedure, I watched the long, transverse belly incision complete its circular orbit. Using a lap pad to follow the scalpel, I wiped away the crimson tears puddling on her abdomen as it wept and counted the layers as we pushed deeper: skin, fat, Camper's fascia, Scarpa's fascia, retract the abdominal muscles, dissect more facia, then a violet mass, the uterus. Before the uterine incision was made, I was handed two suction tips. The red tip, I was instructed, was for blood. The blue tip, on the other hand, would be for amniotic fluid. I waited anxiously as the resident proceeded, the blade pushing through the beefy, muscular organ as I followed with the red tip in my left hand. Then suddenly, a gush of clear, straw-colored fluid, an expulsive wave, volcanic in nature as the pressure released. I lurched forward with my right hand to collect what I could, and immediately following the turbulent stream of amniotic fluid, I saw ... wet hair.

————

As Baby A began to crown, her hair looked the same as Baby B's. Thin, black, stencil sketched and matted to her head haphazardly. She descended just like my professors had described. She was left occiput anterior, or left side facing up, and with the assistance of my attending, I rotated her body to help deliver the first shoulder. It passed with ease, as did the second. She was in fact slippery, but luckily, she was no match for my hands, clenching fervently, compelled mostly by the unpleasant thought of dropping a stranger's newborn.

Newborns are usually graded at minutes one and five on a ten-point scale called the APGAR. It's an acronym standing for Appearance, Pulse, Grimace, Activity, and Respiration. It has been said jokingly that the only kids who obtain a perfect APGAR score are the children of pediatricians because it is nearly impossible, but generally speaking, a higher score in the first few minutes of life is indicative of a healthier baby. Baby A came out mostly pink in appearance, fading ever so gradually from her torso to a dusky shade of blue in her tiny hands and feet. Acrocyanosis, worthy of one point. Her pulse was strong, about 150 beats per minute on the monitor immediately prior to delivery. Two points. She responded to stimulation of the towel with an irritated furrow of her eyebrows as I dried her off. Two points. She had adequate activity, sometimes referred to as muscular tone. One point. Her breathing was somewhat slow and without a robust cry. One point. A total of seven.

I felt proud of myself for this accomplishment—I had delivered a healthy baby girl. Beneath my mask, I smiled and scanned the room for nods of approval, in the process making eye contact with the nurse who had previously been holding mom's left leg. In lieu of reassurance, she looked on in horror, her eyes opening wider and wider, her mouth agape, her slender right index finger pointing back at me. I looked down at Baby A as my heart, in one brisk squeeze, shuttled a bolus of adrenaline to the rest of my body. My stomach sank beneath the floor, and I started to sweat bullets.

Immediately after the birth, I had distributed Baby A's

weight evenly and gingerly over my two hands, my right supporting the back of her head and my left cradling her midsection. As the nurse pierced my soul with her wordless glower, I looked down and saw the baby's arms were no longer suspended in mid-air but had fallen to either side of my right hand, the weight of gravity pulling them to the earth. Her sausage rolls for legs, once held out in tension, had also slumped toward the ground like a wilted plant left out in the sun. At this point, I had no idea what was happening, but I remembered everything that happened next. The pediatrics team was paged emergently. Moments later, a team of at least six people burst in the room. I handed Baby A over to their custody, where she was immediately placed under a warming hood. Her mouth was suctioned, and she was vigorously rubbed for stimulation. I saw a nurse place a stethoscope over her chest and mime out Baby A's heart rate, tapping her index finger into her thumb high over her head for all to bear witness. Tap ... tap ... tap. It shouldn't have been that slow.

A pediatrics resident started performing compressions using two fingers to artificially squeeze Baby A's heart through the chest wall. This lasted at least twenty seconds. While this was happening, from the other side of the room, I overheard my attending speaking to mom in hushed tones, "Your baby is doing fine. You had a small tear that we're going to fix up while they work over there. Everything is going to be okay." I swiveled my head back to the pediatrics side of the room and I heard, "Do you think we need to intubate?" At this point, mom started wailing in distress.

———

Because of the emergent nature of Baby B's procedure, in the haste of the moment, the uterine incision was placed slightly higher than where would have been ideal. The downstream effect of this misplacement was that, for the size of the baby boy (who ended up being well over nine pounds), we had much more difficulty getting him out. After a few failed attempts at pushing him through the uterine incision, the decision was made to put a small vacuum on his head. We would need to hand-pump in a small amount of suction which would in turn afford us the leverage we needed to get him out. This was not an uncommon necessity.

A decent amount of force was required to free him from his confines, but in time, the uterus relinquished its grasp. However, what he left behind was a disaster. In most cases, following delivery, the uterus should reflexively begin to clamp back down, slowly shrinking in size. In the process, it compresses small arteries and veins to help tamponade blood loss. It also helps to expel the placenta, a highly vascular structure in itself. It is analogous to a piece of tape stuck on the outside of an inflated balloon: as one begins to let air out of the balloon (uterus contracting on itself), the tape that was stuck to the balloon (placenta) eventually peels off. For the mom of Baby B, as a result of her prolonged labor, her uterus was having a hard time clamping down. It was fatigued. Her placenta was also in ruins in the sense that it didn't come out in one piece. When we pulled on the umbilical cord, it tore like tissue paper. As a result, open blood vessels were now freely losing blood. By the time the placenta was completely evacuated by hand, mom had lost nearly two liters of blood, roughly 40 percent of a normal human's blood volume.

———

A few moments after the residents had asked about intubation, Baby A let out a fragile cry—she was protecting her airway. The whole room let out a sigh of relief. Just as quickly as she'd gone limp, she was back in mom's arms. We all rejoiced, the color in dad's face returned, and I collected what was left of my dignity. In the heat of the moment, I was, of course, afraid for Baby A's safety. I was also equally worried that, in some way, I was responsible for her sudden decompensation. To my relief, she had made a full recovery. I also listened in on the debrief between the obstetrics team and pediatrics, who were discussing the decision to administer Dilaudid for pain control hours earlier. Apparently, while a potent painkiller, it is not without unintended consequences, given the medication has the potential to cross the placenta and make its way into a fetus' bloodstream. When Baby A came out, she had exhibited side effects from this class of medication including decreased tone and respiratory depression. She had essentially had a transient overdose on narcotics but was now in the resolution phase.

———

The steady bleeding from the mother of Baby B did not resolve as quickly, but in time, hemostasis was achieved. I found out, too, that the blood volume in pregnant women increases significantly in the months prior to delivery to help tolerate significant fluid shifts in the birthing process, and while she had indeed lost enough blood to classify as a postpartum hemorrhage, she was in stable condition, as was her baby boy.

Neither of these two deliveries were textbook—far from it—but at the end of the day, thankfully, both moms were under quality care and their babies, after much fanfare, came out healthy.

In room number twelve, I found myself surrounded by thirteen other people. In OR number two, an entirely separate set of bodies enveloped me. In the chaos of both of these moments, looking at these new sets of parents, I thought about my own, who at my age, were already caring for two small toddlers. My older sister was born when my mom and dad were twenty-two and twenty-three, respectively. Fourteen months later, I popped out. In stories I hear now, they tell me about how difficult this made life. They share tales from a cramped apartment in shady parts of town, how they took on a larger mortgage to get into a better school district. I hear about piling mounds of credit card debt transferred from one card to the next in serial fashion to make ends meet. Nightmares of them trying to find jobs to support their young family, sleepless nights with kids who would not stop crying, who refused to eat the chicken nuggets that they could afford, who were suspended from daycare for getting into fights. The struggle and sacrifices they'd gone through to raise kids as barely adults themselves quite frankly impress and terrify me.

Here I was, twenty-five years old and jobless, still living in an apartment with three other dudes. I had no source of income (quite the opposite, actually); I barely knew what a 401k was and had just heard of the term Roth IRA but had no idea how to manage one. I didn't see myself being responsible enough to care for a child, and I didn't even trust myself with the responsibility of owning a dog. To me, these milestones—settling down and having kids—always seemed so far off. They were points on the horizon that never seemed to be getting any closer. For most of my life, I desperately have *not* wanted a kid, thinking that a baby in the picture, for right or wrong, would ruin my grandiose plans built on the foundation of higher education. Of course, I still believe it will happen at some point, but that future seems so distant. I don't know if I will ever feel ready. For now, wedding invitations are showing up in my mailbox, friends are posting screenshots of ultrasound pictures online, and I am left to ask what memo I must have missed and how it is that they know they're ready. At some point, the nature of marriage and childrearing tipped from predominantly evil to good. The funny thing is nobody ever told me when and how this is supposed to happen, but for others around me, it just sort of did.

In room twelve and in OR two, I looked on at these parents cradling their babies, staring into their eyes as they blinked them open to take in their first look at the world. Each pair of parents admired their baby's beautiful, wrinkly face, petite hands, chubby legs, and the cutest little socks now covering their feet. I took in the expression on dad's face as he wrapped his arms around exhausted mom, who'd spent the past nine months carrying and delivering something they'd created together, something that was inherently a piece of them. Over time, they'd have the privilege of raising this unique being with their own personality and quirks, of watching them grow, of loving them without reservation. Looking on at these parents as they got acquainted with the newest member of their family, the stress and excitement of the previous hours faded away, and for a brief moment in time, all I saw was bliss.

11

JAMAAL

Today I consider myself the luckiest man on the face of this earth.

—Lou Gehrig

DOCTOR-PATIENT INTERACTIONS take place in two main settings. When patients are "admitted," they're sent to the inpatient ward, where they stay overnight. This level of acuity is typically reserved for patients requiring increased supervision in the form of twenty-four-hour nursing staff, heart rate monitors, and easy access to invasive tests and advanced imaging. The outpatient setting, on the other hand, is set up primarily by appointment and is likely representative of the average individual's schema of a doctor's office. It is complete with a front desk attendant, "Say Ahh" moments, and fancy instruments with disposable plastic tips attached to the wall by those characteristic coiling wires. This is where a patient would go for an annual physician visit or to be seen in an urgent care clinic.

A medical student's role in the outpatient setting varies wildly by supervising doctor. Some attendings are relatively hands-on with their patients. In these instances, students are relegated to what amounts to little more than a shadowing experience. They will follow the doctor into the patient room, situate themselves in a corner, and wordlessly observe the subsequent interaction, feigning excitement for this job using nods, soft smiles, and the occasional furrow of the eyebrows as their primary means of communication. With other attendings, students get more autonomy. In these moments, they can see the patients by themselves, apply their knowledge to collect a history, think critically, and provide their own assessments of what they think is afflicting a given individual. In all these outpatient experiences, though, it always felt like a disproportionate amount of my time was dedicated to watching circles change color.

On the scheduling page of the electronic medical record, patients were listed with their presenting complaint. In this tab, on the far-left column of the computer screen next to each patient name, was a small circle whose body was filled in by various colors throughout the day. Over the course of the clinic, as patients were seen and dismissed, these circles would change colors, each associated with a unique connotation. A circle filled in white meant the patient had not yet arrived. A circle filled in yellow meant the patient had arrived and was waiting to be roomed. A circle filled in green meant the patient was ready for the physician to enter. Lastly, a circle filled in black meant the visit was closed and the patient was no longer in-house.

I met Jamaal on my pediatrics rotation shortly after his circle turned green. Because he was twenty-two years old at the time, I was sure he felt out of place meeting me in this setting. I was told he was coming to the pediatrics clinic for the sake of "continuity of care"—he had been seen here as a kid, and the doctors knew him well. The clinic where I worked was also funded by the Center for Medicare & Medicaid Services (CMS), and I could only assume that health insurance coverage played a role in Jamaal's decision as well. At this point in my third year, I found myself in the outpatient setting, performing well-child check-ups, sports physicals, and strep tests for kids in the community. I recognized quickly that this visit would be significantly different than the others—Jamaal's chief complaint was anal warts. Given this presentation, I scrolled through his chart suspecting what I eventually found: human immunodeficiency virus, HIV.

The history of HIV is tumultuous. When HIV first came to the public attention in the 1970s, it was a new disease. Because of its novelty, it was a terrifying diagnosis. What scientists and physicians knew back then was that it predominantly affected men who have sex with men (MSM) as well as injection drug users (due to what we would later learn was sexual transmission and/or contact with infected blood). For this reason, the disease was heavily stigmatized, initially called gay-related immune deficiency (GRID). As the scientific community learned more about this virus, early reports linked it to a variety of seemingly disjointed and, frankly, confusing conditions but, ultimately, for most patients it ended the same way. In September of 1982, the Centers for Disease Control and Prevention (CDC) recognized AIDS as an official disease state. As most are aware, this is a deadly condition.

HIV is what is called a retrovirus. Retroviruses are all equipped with a special enzyme called a reverse transcriptase.

While the majority of viruses replicate their genetic material (ribonucleic acid [RNA] in most cases) directly in the host cell's cytoplasm, retroviruses use reverse transcriptase to reproduce their RNA in the form of deoxyribose nucleic acid (DNA, the genetic material in humans). This is unusual because the Central Dogma of Molecular Biology explicitly describes the flow of genetic information in cells as beginning with DNA, followed by transcription into RNA, and lastly, translation into proteins, which drive most functions within cells, the building blocks of all living things.

HIV violates this fundamental principal with its reverse transcriptase by converting RNA not into proteins but instead into DNA, allowing it to directly incorporate into a host's genetic material. Once incorporated, a host is then tricked into thinking the new viral DNA is part of its own genetic makeup. It then starts making additional copies of the virus on its own. It's a brilliant system, espionage for viruses.

Over time, as the virus continues to replicate, it causes the brunt of its destruction indirectly by reducing the number of helper T cells, or CD4 lymphocytes, the cells responsible for our acquired immunity. This does not kill a host, but the consequences of this action are fatal. Without a robust immune response, opportunistic infections like pneumocystis carinii pneumonia (PCP), human herpesvirus 8 (HHV8, the virus responsible for Kaposi's sarcoma), human papillomavirus (HPV), and others go unchecked, often ending in death. In an immunocompetent individual without HIV, the immune system usually swiftly recognizes these infections and rarely allows them to flourish.

Many modern HIV drugs, called antiretrovirals, target the most upstream of all of these issues: the reverse transcriptase enzyme. Without the cloak of reverse transcriptase for HIV, there is no subsequent destruction of CD4 lymphocytes, no immunodeficiency, and no proliferation of opportunistic infections. In today's world, because of these remarkable new drugs, HIV is no longer a death sentence.

But anal warts were a symptom of HPV which, to me, indicated that something was off. My attending was aware of this, and prior to my entering the room, he had asked me to inquire about Jamaal's medication regimen. Jamaal, to his credit, did not withhold information and answered my questions without hesitation. He explained that, since his diagnosis of HIV a little more than a year ago, he had refused antiretroviral medication. When I asked why this might be the case, he answered that, for the most part, this decision had been out of fear: in his mind, the very act of taking a medication was an admission that he had a chronic and potentially debilitating condition. He had seen many cases of HIV in his community, and he knew that the outlook could be bleak. For this reason, he avoided the medications we offered and the admission to himself of the severity of his new identity.

To me, a patient with a relatively new diagnosis of Crohn's disease, this was an internal conflict with which I was acutely familiar. When first diagnosed, I faced a similar decision. As a medical student, I had read in textbooks and seen in person the presentation of Crohn's disease and how it could wreak havoc on the human form through a diverse arsenal of weapons. For the past three years, I had, in fact, scrubbed into multiple operations where we sought to remove large segments of the bowel affected by stricturing disease. These patients, in each instance, were close to my age and, coincidentally, patients of my personal gastroenterologist, who had recommended this same exact procedure to me just weeks prior to my general surgery rotation.

I later took care of a Crohn's patient affected by a recto-vaginal fistula, an abnormal connection between the rectum and vagina such that the repeated assault of fecal matter on the sensitive lining of the vaginal wall had created a raw tract, leaving in its place an opioid use dependency as the primary method of pain control. I met yet another patient who had been to the ED over fifty times in two years because of recurrent bowel obstruction episodes. I even had a resident tell me that Crohn's disease was on his list of "Top Five Worst Non-Cancerous Diseases," not knowing that I carried the diagnosis myself.

The decision for me to start taking a biologic therapy, a class of medication reserved only for the most advanced cases of Crohn's disease, was not about the medication. It was, like for Jamaal, about what the medication represented: that there was an autoimmune disease for which we have no cure and with which I was afflicted. I did not reveal this commonality to him at the time, but in not so many words, I did attempt to articulate how I understood where he was coming from. That, yes, the act of taking a medication was potentially an acknowledgement that there was something serious affecting his body, but at the same time, it could be a liberating decision insofar as it allowed him to take back power over his disease.

By the end of this visit, many things had happened:

- My perspective had resonated with Jamaal, and he agreed to start taking antiretroviral therapy.
- He had felt comfortable enough with me during our

conversation to also talk about his spirituality and the intersection with his sexuality.

- During my review of systems, a basic series of questions querying other potential symptoms a patient might be experiencing, I had a growing suspicion that he might also have been presenting with new-onset diabetes. For this reason, I advocated that we order a series of labs, which ultimately confirmed this diagnosis as well.

- The visit culminated with Jamaal asking me to use his iPhone to take a picture of his anus so that he could better appreciate the warts that had brought him into the office in the first place.

- We scheduled a return visit for one week from that day so that we could check in on his initiation of antiretroviral therapy. I was excited because I was still on service next week, and I would see him once more before leaving the rotation. I left the clinic that day the highest I had ever felt in all of medical school after a patient interaction.

In all of this, I felt like I was finally doing good in the world. I was *doctoring*. I had made somebody else's life better; I had helped make somebody feel more comfortable, less scared; I had put into place all of the skills I had been learning over the past three years to communicate a complicated medical diagnosis and treatment plan; I had even diagnosed my patient with a condition from which he had no complaints on arrival but which, over time, had the potential to slowly pathologize his heart, kidneys, and eyes, among other vital organs. In Jamaal, I could see the pieces coming together in my own learning and path to becoming a doctor. All of these small moments had finally built into something grand. This encounter really felt like a testament to how far I had come, and I think that is why it stuck with me even after I left the clinic that day.

The next week, when Jamaal arrived, he recognized me immediately. In the brief fifteen minutes allotted for his visit, we caught up and shared a few laughs over small talk and casual conversation. I learned that he had initiated his regimen, bought a pill box, and had set up reminders on his phone so he would not forget his daily dose. He had been supported in this decision by his friends and a few family members and felt confident with this new path he had set out for himself.

Of course, a week after I first met Jamaal, I actually learned that I didn't work in Hollywood; rather, I worked in a clinic on Cottage Grove and 55th Street. The truth was that, the next week when I showed up for work, I took a seat in the back office and watched Jamaal's circle. I watched it pop up when his appointment came, outlined in black and filled in white. I watched it stay white as his assigned time came and went, even after I hovered by reception hoping to see him waltz through the door. I watched it persist as I stayed late after clinic, saying to myself that he would eventually show up and we would squeeze him in.

After the lights turned off, his circle eventually went from white to black without the yellow or green in between, and I walked home that night perhaps the lowest I ever felt after a patient non-interaction. On this walk, I realized that this feeling wasn't anything novel. There were a lot of inconsistencies within medicine in which I had played some part over the past few years. Whether it was patient noncompliance to their pharmacotherapy, structural barriers to care and access, or more generally, the broken, patchwork nature of our healthcare system, I knew patients could fall through the cracks at any number of places on their journeys from sickness to health.

I'd like to think the reason Jamaal never showed up was because the traffic that day was especially bad, or that his boss wouldn't let him out of work in a timely manner, or that maybe he was babysitting or caring for a family member. But as I worked later that year in the ED and saw patients with chronic conditions presenting for the first time with horrible manifestations of preventable diseases, I could not help but think of Jamaal and how what likely happened on that Wednesday a week after we first met was that he just did not want to come back. He was a young man who was scared and maybe didn't know what he wanted or even forgot. And then, on the day when he was supposed to return to clinic, all the progress that I thought we'd made wasn't enough to overcome the fear, the anxiety, and maybe the apathy. I think this was, and is, difficult for me to process because I had experienced this profoundly intimate interaction with a stranger and never got to see him again. I cannot imagine many other people have taken a picture of his bare bottom, and I probably know more about him than most other people in his life, all from a fifteen-minute interaction. It's hard to not get even a glimmer of closure from this encounter. It's hard to not want more for Jamaal and the future "Jamaals" I know I'll meet throughout my career.

In all the highs and lows of patient care, I still feel like the luckiest man on the face of this earth—that I get to wake up each day and do this job. In time, though, I have learned that it comes with the understanding that I can't fix every problem that walks through the door, no matter how badly I desire to do so. Sometimes, the circles never change colors, and what else can we do when this happens but sit in the workroom waiting, staring, and hoping that it turns green, letting us know that our patient has arrived and is waiting to be seen?

12

FOOTPRINTS

No one ever told me that grief felt so like fear.

—C.S. Lewis, *A Grief Observed*

TEN LITTLE DOTS hovered delicately over symmetric arches, as if suspended in midair. Tiptoes inked in jet-black, matching in color and in the pattern of intricate swirls, the heels now plastered onto a brilliant yellow backdrop. There they stood in time and space, the smallest footprints I had ever seen in my life, a now permanent fixture stamped on a piece of cardboard, transferred by the hands of a nurse attempting to conceal the noiseless commotion of tears welling up then rolling down the contours of her fog-free, foam, fluid-resistant surgical mask.

I had seen this before; how could I forget that queer shade of yellow? Each iteration prior, it had been accompanied by the phrase *WELCOME TO THE WORLD* emblazoned across the top.

This time, there was a barely perceptible diagonal cut just below where the words would have been, the only remnant of the hasty trimming that had happened just a moment ago.

My patient, who would receive this memento, was a thirty-two-year-old G1P0 at twenty-two weeks.[i]

Before meeting her, I had skimmed her electronic medical record, looking for any details that could have prepared me for the upcoming procedure. I learned of a history of infertility conquered by the advances of modern medicine. After multiple rounds of in vitro fertilization, a confirmatory transvaginal ultrasound had informed her that she had succeeded. Several months later, however, a routine second trimester body scan revealed the unimaginable: her baby boy had bilateral cleft lips and a large cardiac defect along with a host of other abnormalities. The official diagnosis was a chromosomal deletion that even her doctors had yet to fully comprehend. Regardless of our understanding of the specifics of her baby's condition, the outcome remained unchanged: the fetus would not be viable. Management at this gestational age, I read, was dilation and evacuation.

Here was where our paths overlapped: an expectant mother at the juncture of perhaps the most difficult time in her life and a medical student on week two of two of his labor and delivery rotation. With her H&P fresh in mind, I entered the operating room, greeted by a host of familiarities. To my left, a scrub nurse sorted an impressive collection of silver-plated tools. Another tallied the number of open sponges on a dry-erase board. One,

---

[i]   In obstetrics, "G" stands for "gravida" which means the total number of times a woman has been pregnant, while "P" stands for "para" which indicates the number of times a woman has carried that pregnancy to term.

two, three, four, five. One, two, three, four, five. Toward the far wall, an anesthesiologist combed through a tangle of wires and tethered the loose ends to machines beeping methodically in the background. From behind me, the attending physician and chief resident arrived with hands high, purified water dripping down flexed elbows onto the grainy floor below. They donned their sterile uniforms, and a nurse stepped forward to first secure the Velcro straps around their necks, then tie off the gowns with a hurried knot at the waist.

Normally, I find comfort in these rituals, the predictability of each player and their respective routines. While this ballet was no different in choreography, the rigidity with which it was executed suggested a degree of fragility that was almost precious, as if even the slightest misstep would tip it off its axis. I stepped to the side and anchored myself in the ground, focusing on the center of the room, where our patient lay unconscious, hair pulled back under the confines of a bouffant cap, hands clenched tightly across her chest.

For the rest of the procedure, I stood behind the bodies of the attending physician and resident, peering around oversized gowns and past four hands in the narrowest of spaces, shifting my gaze from liquid red over solid blue to the black and white of the monitor, those hazy reflections of soundwaves bouncing off surgical instruments and fetal tissue. The blur of colors served as but a canvas for other images now burned into my memory like a flip book connecting one moment in time to another.

I had been warned this would be a challenging case both technically and emotionally. Because of this, I was not surprised by the surgeon's hands, steady as they were, struggling to perform their task; I was not alarmed when tenaculums slipped from their clamped position on her cervix or when Hegars titrated at a slower rate than anticipated. Still, no amount of preparation could have removed the sinking feeling as I watched one being crumple emotionally and another physically. No preface could have prevented a mental trip to a week prior, mint chocolate chip in hand at a fountain in the middle of town, where a black Labrador roamed carelessly, and children splashed about in laughter. I looked on as a boy chased his sister into a pool of water, slipped, and careened through the air as if in slow motion. From my seat, I flinched under the impulse to do something—anything—to foil the inevitable. How do you intervene when there is nothing that can be done to save them? How do you communicate to somebody else that you are with them?

A stitch was placed. An hour had passed since the blade was requested. Whispers went around the room. The yellow piece of cardboard was ushered. She was a thirty-two-year-old G1P0.

Words fail to describe the anguish one must feel to have life taken from them. I was only seeing it from the other side: the purest look of fear as the anesthesia was metabolized two then three then four half-lives, an event horizon that, like a supernatural force, devoured not just all happiness, but sadness and anger from the room until all that was left was a somber emotionless silence that sapped the breath out of my own lungs, stole even the wandering from my gaze, which fixed straight ahead at what was wholly important in that moment and simultaneously something of newly nothingness. It is in this setting that we attempt to perform little gestures: I find myself running to gather warm blankets, stretching out my arm to reach for her hand, placing two little black footprints that will never grow any bigger atop pleated sheets, now immortalized on a yellow backdrop. I want so viscerally to be able to do more. Sometimes in medicine, this is the most we can do.

Despite all our technology, collective experience, the papers decorating our office walls, and the letters after our names, there are times when even the most seasoned veteran has no more to offer than the trainee. While we cannot fix everybody, we must still ascribe importance to every action we take. Sometimes, all we can give within the context of another's care is our time, our emotional energy, and these gestures which, though small in nature, can carry profound meaning.

Just two little feet. Jet-black on a yellow background. The smallest footprints I had ever seen in my life. Placed atop the gurney as my patient was wheeled out of the operating room and into recovery, in every sense of the word.

13

EVA

At a cardiac arrest, the first procedure is to take your own pulse.

—Samuel Shem, "Law Number III," *The House of God*

Eva was an eighty-seven-year-old with suspected heart failure. She arrived on the floor hooked up to four liters of oxygen delivered to her nose by a plastic tube called a nasal cannula. When I introduced myself to her, she offered an earnest look of confusion in place of traditional hellos. She was able to state her name but had no idea about where she was, the present year, nor what had brought her into the hospital. Because she could not answer my questions, I proceeded instead with the physical exam.

Her neck veins were engorged and pulsed rhythmically under my scrutiny. I could hear her lungs crackle with each inspiration as I placed a stethoscope over the backside of her brittle ribcage. From the front, her heart plodded along with a harsh systolic murmur out of the mitral window, and the skin overlying her scaly shins was tense and boggy. Each finding served as a clue hinting at the presence of "volume overload," or fluid outside of the vasculature—when the heart is either unable to squeeze with adequate fervor or relax appropriately before each new beat, blood may pool in various places, forcing water and other solvents like plasma into the soft tissue. The lungs were a common site, as were the legs.

As part of our workup, we searched for evidence in support of our theory by collecting labs: a basic metabolic panel, a brain natriuretic peptide (BNP) level, a cardiac enzyme level, a chest X-ray, and an electrocardiogram, or ECG for short. We discovered that her creatinine, a marker for kidney function, was higher than the normal range, suggesting decreased renal perfusion, which could have been caused by blood not flowing forward briskly enough to allow the kidneys to filter effectively (because of a failing heart, for instance). Her BNP was significantly elevated, and her troponins were in the 250s, offering a mixed picture between potential heart failure and a myocardial infarction, also known as a heart attack. On her chest X-ray, her lungs were diffusely white, confirming the presence of fluid, which likely contributed to her increased work of breathing and new oxygen requirement. We treated this with a thoracentesis on hospital day number one, a procedure requiring a large-bore needle to be threaded into the lung space, under the auspices of continuous ultrasound in many cases, with the goal of draining fluid. The proceduralists had to be careful here to not puncture, and subsequently collapse, the fragile bag of air in the process.

We further started her on intravenous Lasix, a medication that encouraged the loss of water by inhibiting its resorption in the kidneys. The theory was that, by increasing the amount of urine Eva produced, she would slowly start to dry out, and her tired heart's workload would lighten. Her doctors believed that, in time, this approach would lead to an improvement in her symptoms. This was, after all, the classic management of heart failure.

As the days passed one after the other, Eva's condition didn't improve as we'd hoped. Her lungs kept reaccumulating fluid even after we took off more than 1.7 liters of transudate (clear, watery fluid that leaks out of blood vessels when there's a pressure or protein imbalance in the body, such as in heart or liver disease); her legs continued to grow more edematous no matter how much we diuresed with Lasix; her kidney function declined; she barely ate. By the end of the first week, she no longer knew who she was.

———

When I moved to Chicago, like any poor graduate student, my roommates and I filled our apartment with furniture from Ikea. On the way out, I stopped by the houseplant section, a miniature ficus catching my eye. It was a gorgeous plant with a magnificent skeleton, filled out at the top with a hundred little waxy leaves coated in deep emerald. Its trunk plunged into the soil at two places, the main stalks coiling around each other as they corkscrewed into the earth. It came in a modern white planter, and I knew it had to be mine. I placed it on my nightstand when I got home and watered it on a strict schedule. Over the next few months, every now and then after class, I would come home only to discover that a new leaf had fallen to the floor. The tree was otherwise healthy enough that I couldn't tell from where it had fallen, but it had fallen, nonetheless. Over time, this process repeated itself slowly until, all at once, I realized there were only a few leaves left.

In psychology, the concept of the just-noticeable difference, or Weber's Law, describes the notion that there is a fixed threshold between two stimuli required to detect a real difference. Below this threshold, slight disparities between two stimuli go unnoticed; only when above this value can they be appreciated. If the initial stimulus happened to be the weight of an object, for example, and Weber's constant for weight was specifically found to be two percent, a 100-pound barbell would *feel* the same as a 101-pound barbell despite their being different weights. If the weight were instead increased to 102 pounds, the two repetitions would now *feel* appreciably different. In both scenarios, the weights were, in all actuality, different, but the difference was only detected once above the Weber constant value. This principle can be applied to any two stimuli and would receive a different Weber constant: noise level, specific shades of red, object dimensions, even the number of leaves on a given tree.

For Eva and many other hospitalized patients, the experience of dying, while inherently more complex than this psychological principle, shares fundamental similarities with Weber's Law. Looking back now, it is easy to see that Eva was getting worse, ever so slightly each day. Her appetite all but went away, her oxygen requirement increased from four to six liters, her mean arterial pressure dropped incrementally. In the moment though, most days when I checked in on her, she seemed more or less the same—the daily depreciation that she *truly* experienced was below my just-noticeable difference threshold. While her minute changes in function, perceived or not, were not enough to necessitate a more aggressive management strategy, a week and a day after her hospital admission, she had depreciated enough for me to finally recognize how bad her condition had become. She was dying.

———

The spectrum of death in the hospital varies wildly. Some patients ask for all life-sustaining therapeutics, while others prefer to take a more conservative approach. Some go quickly, and others experience a more protracted and indolent course. In the ED, we see a lot of the quick cases. They often come in on a stretcher via emergency medical services, having been found in the midst of a heart attack, after a gunshot or other penetrating wound, or status post fall from great heights. On arrival, they are immediately shuttled to the trauma bay, where a team of providers stand at the ready to perform cardiopulmonary resuscitation (CPR), push epinephrine, and direct other lifesaving heroics.

CPR requires chest compressions to mechanically squeeze the heart, ideally delivered at a rate of 100–120 beats per minute. While one provider performs compressions, another helps secure the airway and delivers oxygen to the lungs via a bag valve mask. Compressions last for cycles two minutes in duration, after which the team will pause, check for a pulse, and deliver a shock to the heart, if indicated, prior to resuming compressions. The codes that I had witnessed usually lasted at least three rounds before our efforts were determined to be fruitless.

In other settings, patients often went more slowly, over the course of weeks to months. These cases were arguably more difficult to watch because these particular patients offered a glimpse into who they were as people, what they valued, and what their lives were like outside of the hospital. I met a woman on my psychiatry rotation who suffered from a rare vascular disease called polyarteritis nodosa, PAN for short. She came to the office looking for help managing new symptoms of depression related to her diagnosis. In the course of our initial evaluation, we had asked a series of questions to better understand the symptoms she was experiencing. We learned that it had been about a year since she had received her diagnosis of PAN. She had been told that there was no cure for this inflammatory vasculitis and that the aggressive nature of the disease meant she did not have long to live. In time, no matter how much medication she was offered or consumed, there was little that could be done to attenuate the slow and painful assault on her kidneys. They would soon fail, and she would expire not long after that.

Many patients afflicted with fatal diseases say it is inexplicably difficult to find a community. Family and friends, and even psychiatrists, can offer support but are unable to fully empathize with the plight of those carrying the burden of a diagnosis, and more importantly, how that diagnosis might alter their lives. For this reason, many patients look to support groups with others who share similar diagnoses for processing and coping with being *sick*. Because PAN was extraordinarily rare, we had asked whether she had been successful in finding a community of other PAN patients through support groups, either in person or online. She told us she had, in fact, looked to find others through Facebook, joining numerous groups dedicated to connecting individuals affected by PAN. She shared that, despite gaining entry into these established groups, she grew more discouraged and more depressed by this endeavor, as every time she connected with somebody whose story resonated with her or with whom she felt like she could have a genuine conversation, she would reach out with a direct message only to later learn that they had already passed away.

———

I called Eva's daughter early in the admission to get a better sense of who she was at baseline. Her daughter explained that, outside of the hospital, her mom was vivacious. Eva had indeed lived a full life, but her daughter was convinced she was not done living. She found it hard to believe that the person I was describing over the phone was the same person she had visited just days prior. She told me about how, even now, at the ripe age of eighty-seven, Eva was still traveling the world, delivering lectures to large audiences. When she wasn't touring the world, she liked to knit, listen to the radio, and spend time with her grandchildren. Sadly, her husband had recently passed away, and since then, she too had experienced a precipitous decline in functional status, which ultimately put her in the hospital. For Eva, the patient I had come to know did not represent the person she was. I knew this to be true and was aware of this, but it was often hard to separate the person from the patient because all I saw from Eva each day was her at her worst, at her most scared, at her least comfortable.

By the end of my second week taking care of Eva, she had earned an official diagnosis: Takotsubo cardiomyopathy, perhaps better known as broken heart syndrome, stress cardiomyopathy, or apical ballooning syndrome. Medically, it is defined as a transient regional systolic dysfunction of the left ventricle, but in layman's terms, it meant a specific region of her heart responsible for pumping blood to the rest of her body was not functioning properly. We suspected it was Takotsubo by the characteristic features of the heart on ultrasound—its "apical balloon" curiously looked like an octopus. But more interestingly, broken heart syndrome gets its namesake from the etiology of the condition. It was thought that this particular type of cardiac disease was caused by increased catecholamine (stress hormone) release, often induced by a significant stress response. In many cases, the stress response was triggered by the loss of a loved one, Eva's husband in this case. About 90 percent of cases occurred in women, and in younger women, this condition was often self-resolving within four weeks. For Eva and other women greater than seventy years old, though, with a known stressor and a decreased ejection fraction, the likelihood of acute heart failure was significantly higher.

I eventually moved on to a new rotation and had to relinquish care for Eva. Her treatment had not changed much since she had arrived and likely would not change much for quite some time, save for a remarkable recovery in heart function. Her disposition would likely include transfer to a nursing home, if she were lucky enough to leave the hospital, where caretakers would be able to watch after her closely without inpatient care's requirements and therefore expenses. There, she might experience a restoration of heart function, or more likely, her condition would continue to depreciate until her heart stopped working altogether. This is, of course, entirely speculation. Modern medicine has gotten a lot better at prolonging the end stages of life. It can cover up major deficits with shiny machines and new medication formulations specially designed in one way or another to help the heart pump stronger, to help patients breathe when they are unable to on their own, and to generally ward off death. At a certain point, though, it can no longer hold off the inevitable and patients eventually move on, sometimes after a few rounds of CPR and others with the pulling of a plug.

————

In the face of death, I've surprised myself at my newfound resilience. In the violence of intubations and defibrillations, in the organized chaos of screaming the Glasgow Coma Scale, in shouting medication orders, and in counting the two minutes passing before a shock must be delivered, I was initially convinced it must have all built up to something spectacular. Shortly after the last round of compressions ceased, and well before the patient was zipped into a large bag, just as quickly as doctors, nurses, and technicians had gathered, they dispersed back to their regular nooks. On the way, they cracked jokes about an Instagram Reel they had scrolled past earlier in the day or about the patient's unorthodox tattoos.

The first time my resident pronounced the time of death, I was stunned by the lack of ceremony. After the second, then third, then fourth code of the night, the picture started to make more sense. The first responders on the scene, participating in their 402nd, 403rd, and 404th codes didn't actually know these patients at all. Each simply represented an opportunity to do their job, and the reality for them, more often than not, was that this aspect of their job was not that successful. Despite what movies and TV shows make it out to be, CPR is only about 10 percent effective. Patients dying on the table was the norm and not the exception, so when a person did not miraculously wake up from chest compressions, while discouraging, it wasn't new or surprising. Likewise, to a physician who has dealt with death for decades, even the story of somebody dying of PAN represented more of a trope than an individual story of tragedy.

Whether in the ED, the psych clinic, or the small room housing Eva, the way these scenarios played out reminded me of a December afternoon during MS3. At the 47th Street stop, I waited for a Red Line train to take me up north into the city. The station is situated, peculiarly, in the middle of Interstate 90, such that cars whizz past on either side at speeds of up to eighty miles per hour. From my perch, I watched a car in the northbound lanes round the gentle curve, spin out, career into the median, and flip over, taking out a few others before sliding to a halt. Soon after, police were on the scene beginning to block off the three leftmost lanes, allowing a narrow stream of cars to trickle through the far-right lanes. Anxiously, I watched how, one by one, each car caught in traffic filtered past in series, impatiently throwing on their blinker and cutting off the person behind them in their passage forward. Through the windshields, I could see them slow down to peek at the wreckage before moving on with their lives, seemingly otherwise unaffected.

In debriefing with residents in the ED, with my co-students on the rotation, with my roommates over dinner, I knew I was not alone. Sooner rather than later, these conversations would no longer be the first thing we'd discuss when we got home, even though it hadn't changed the fact that the illness or injury was likely the worst thing that had ever happened to each of our patients. We'd push forward, I think, because it was not our job to cry over our patients, though this may happen. It *was* our job, however, to receive patients at their most vulnerable and least human, to accept them, to help them feel safe, to comfort them, to care for them, and to be there with them when they needed us. Unfortunately, we could not do this for another patient if we were still carrying the last with us.

———

Late one night, I spoke with my then-girlfriend and now wife, Sarah, about this topic. Over the course of our clinical rotations, we tried to better understand the suffering around us and where our emotional compartmentalizing fit into this process. In response, she told me a story about a character named Charon. In Greek mythology, she told me, there were five rivers of the Underworld, ruled over by Hades. Among these, the Acheron was the most prominent and noteworthy, serving as the physical barrier between the mortal world and the afterlife. It was this river that the living could not cross on their own to enter the Underworld and which, likewise, the dead could not traverse back across to rejoin the living.

When the Greeks died, a psychopomp, or spiritual guide— like Hermes or Thanatos (God of Death)—of the newly deceased, would be at the ready to deliver souls to the bank of the Acheron. Waiting there for them would be Charon. Charon served Hades in his role as the Ferryman of the Dead, shepherding individuals across the Acheron in exchange for a fee, a single obol coin. As a result, the loved ones of the Greeks often left an offering atop the eyelids or in the mouths of the dead to serve as this token, such that they could avoid the alternate punishment of roaming the earthly shores of the Acheron for 100 years. It was thought that the poor souls unable to pay Charon his wage gave rise to ghosts as they wandered aimlessly, waiting to cross over to their final resting place.

Early characterizations of Charon were not kind. He was

often depicted as a gruesome character with a foul scent. He had a long, unkempt beard which covered a grimace, weathered by generations of heavy winds encountered on his journey to-and-fro. He wore ragged garbs and held a long boatman's pole in one hand, which he allegedly used to beat his passengers. In later depictions, his eyes were made of fire; he had wings and wielded hammers; and he was, at times, even sketched as a living skeleton or grim reaper of sorts. For all this attention to his physical appearance, he was often a peripheral character in the Greek myths, appearing only at the ending of a tragedy or at a hero's untimely demise. Not much is stated about his emotions or views toward his own profession.

Sometimes, Sarah told me that she thought about those boat rides. She wondered about whether Charon was immune to the pain and suffering of the souls he ferried to a new shore. She wondered if he let them tell him about their lives, if he entertained stories of their wishes and their desires, their unfulfilled and fulfilled dreams. On the days when she would come home from the hospital after a long shift only to submerge herself in the sheets, hoping to discard all memories of the day, she would think that he must be an impassive figure, callous to their strife. But on those rare Chicago winter mornings, when the sunshine peeked through the gray and sent streaks of red-orange across the sky, in the quiet of the snow which dusted the ground, she would remember that there was something as beautiful as the warmth of the rays on her skin, and in these moments, the world would feel bright again. In these moments, she would realize that he had to care, that as he guided souls from one realm into the next, from their earthly tethers to their unearthly home, that he had to concern himself with their stories, for their stories were what made him who he was.

14

PANDEMIC

One day, right, we will go out to a cafe with a friend and then sit in a cinema and what would have once been a totally mundane afternoon will now be the most wonderful experience. We will be aware of all the luck we never saw.

—Matt Haig

January 16

JINU

Late March New York City trip. Sean is free then to come visit. Austin, please come thru.

AUSTIN

I'm down.

February 29

GEORGIA (SISTER)

First death from corona in US.

> Disliked "First death from corona in US."

March 6

AUSTIN

Sean, what's your take on all this coronavirus shit?

JINU

I'm not Sean butttttt it's gonna die down. It's not worse than the flu? There's so much misinformation going around.

> I guess it depends on your metric for worse. People are freaking out now bc it's a new strain and nobody knows the exact number affected. So far it's worse than the flu in terms of mortality (2% vs. 0.1%) but obv not as many people are affected comparatively.

> Idk I feel like xenophobia is playing a role in the hysteria but death rate and how its targeting old people isn't encouraging. Also seems like it's not at its worst point yet so tbd how bad it gets.

AUSTIN

I'm assuming everything is still good for next weekend tho? Is NYC like shut down or anything?

JINU

We are still good. Honestly the city hasn't done anything yet. They just want people to wash their hands.

I'm a little concerned. There's a nonzero chance we gotta quarantine after going. Schools are shutting down, my conference just got cancelled, people are losing their minds at the hospital.

March 9

Google search

"Rudy Gobert microphone incident"

———

GEORGIA

Fulton County schools closed down. Teacher tested positive.

March 11

Boys this situation is wild. Apparently mortality in Italy is 20% for patients over 80 yrs old. They stopped giving respiratory support to people over 50 because they don't have resources.

The CDC is projecting the situation in the US is going to be worse than Italy in 11 days.

JINU

Holy fuck…how bad is it in Chicago?

AUSTIN

I saw they cancelled the St. Paddy's Day thing and I know that's usually a big deal. Nothing has really been cancelled in Raleigh but it's obviously much lower density.

I don't think it's that bad yet. Some confirmed cases but I think everyone is expecting it to get worse. School cancelled all meetings >100 people so graduation, match day, revisit, and lectures have been shut down.

March 12
Google search
"Tom Hanks"

March 13

SARAH (GIRLFRIEND)

I think I just found a bedbug.

What? Did it bite you?

SARAH

I heard that DCAM [Duchossois Center for Advanced Medicine] has them. It was crawling on the sheets.

You sure it wasn't a gnat? Maybe came in yesterday when the windows were open so might not be one?

SARAH

sends picture

Fuuuuck.

Ok some not-so-great news. The Ellis
household may or may not but definitely does
have at least 1 bedbug, which most likely
means the call rooms in the hospital have
bedbugs (and/or I am transporting them around
Hyde Park). I put in an order to see if we can
have our apartment inspected but in the
meantime probs want to check for bites on your
person/bugs in your sheets. Will keep everyone
posted :(

RYAN

Well shit.

JASON

Oh boy.

———

SARAH

Hello! The extermination company confirmed
via photo that it IS a bedbug so they want us to
get started on treatments ASAP. In order to get
treatments, we need to prep the house and
arrange to leave during the treatments. They
sent us a checklist of things that have to be
done before a treatment.

Can we do this before tomorrow?

TESS

Just talked to Kathy. Nice lady haha. She said
we need three treatments no matter what. After
the first treatment the guy will tell us if we can
put our clothes back in the closet. If he says
yes, we can do that. If no, then they have to
stay in bags or be cleaned again.

MAYA

So next steps: 1) buying mattress covers 2) putting all clothes into sealed bags 3) taking down all decorations.

March 14

SARAH

Fwd: "While inspecting and treating the unit there were no visible signs of bedbugs observed at time of service."

^!!!!

sends GIF of Tom Brady screaming "Let's Go"

How I feel about the bedbug sitch:

@KColbin on Twitter: "Here's the thing about flattening the curve. It only works if we take the necessary measures before they seem necessary. And if it works, people will think we over-reacted. We have to be willing to look like we overreacted."

———

Hey y'all sorry I have to cancel. NYC is too close to the outbreak...

JINU

What a crazy time to be alive. No worries at all. Sorry for the delay in messaging back I've been sorting all my jobs, labs, and classes the past couple of days.

I'm moving back to Georgia. I don't have a
steady income anymore and my parents want
me back. Research is on hold and there isn't
really anything left for me in NYC. They have a
city-wide lockdown. It sucks but it makes
sense.

———

Google search
"Breonna Taylor"

March 15
Email shared from Harvard Medical School
"In the ICU and ED, as of today, it is now considered counter-
productive to have students on the team. ... Just as many services
are sending some faculty and residents home to stay healthy to
preserve them to be ready to come back when they will soon be
needed, we want to preserve the ways that you as students may
also be able to contribute in important ways. We are therefore
now asking all students, effective immediately, to not come into
clinical rotations for the next week until Sunday March 22nd. ...
We will be reaching out to you as soon as possible regarding
opportunities to return to help provide care in clinical spaces as
these opportunities materialize."

———

Poll in class GroupMe
Do you think that Pritzker should generally be taking the same approach as Harvard?
66.2% YES
33.8% NO

————

Email from dean of students
"Thanks for reaching out. These are rather uncertain times: we are dealing with something new, and things are changing pretty rapidly. For now, the message to your colleagues should be to stay on service unless the teams locally find reason to believe there's rationale to remove you from care. In many ways, these are principles that have been in place all along."

March 16
Email on behalf of general surgery clerkship director
"Hello, you are to go home effective immediately. If you have an oral exam later today, Tuesday, or Wednesday and the faculty have not set it up with you remotely, then we will need to figure that out later. If you are set to do an exam remotely, that is good. But, for now, head home and look for my emails. Thank you."

————

Just got sent home. Clerkship cancelled for the rest of the week. All elective surgery cases cancelled too. The hospital has a really odd energy right now.

Email from dean of students

"With the extension of the University of Chicago spring break, students will be affected as follows:

- MS1 will be managed remotely. Spring quarter will commence on April 6th and your course directors will be reaching out to you with revised syllabi and specific instructions regarding course requirements.
- The MS2 class will also proceed with their study block and scholarship & discovery experience remotely.
- MS3 students should plan to return to their clerkships on Monday, April 6th following the extended spring break. We will be monitoring the situation in the hospitals and will have updates for you regarding any changes in the structure of the clerkship prior to your return.
- MS4 students who are scheduled to return on April 1st for clinical work, you should await further instructions for how required clinical experiences will be managed."

March 17

MOM

shared article

"There are four ways," the doctor told The Daily Beast, "One, it peters out with the weather. Two everybody gets infected, so it's got no new places to go ... so it ends—but that's a pretty horrible ending. Three is a vaccine, which is about a year away. Fourth way is the most likely: we're going to have a few drugs, within a few weeks to a few months, that prevent people from getting infected—like PrEP for HIV—and for treatment."

This doctor is William Haseltine, president of the Global Health think tank ACCESS Health International, who recently chaired the U.S. - China Health Summit in Wuhan, where the virus likely originated.

March 18

GEORGIA

shared article

"Chicago's Midway Airport closed its control tower after 3 technicians tested positive for the coronavirus."

———

MARY KATE

Are you still in school?

Nah rotations are cancelled. I'm pretty worried. I think a lot of people are going to die because of this. It's really serious.

MARY KATE

Wait I'm actually really curious on your take.
People will die because hospitals are
overwhelmed or just generally in terms of how
much the disease will spread?

> Trending towards the ICU's being filled with
> COVID patients in respiratory distress. We won't
> have enough vents to keep all of them alive so
> many COVID patients and patients who
> otherwise wouldn't die from other conditions
> won't have vents. That's what's happening in
> Italy and Spain already.

MARY KATE

What do you think is the proper response? I'm
assuming Sydney [Australia] is a few weeks
behind the US.

> We need more tests because people are going
> around spreading it like mad not knowing they
> have it. I think we need the government to shut
> down everything. Mask mandate. The works.

MARY KATE

It's a hard ask to shut down all businesses. I
definitely agree that human lives are more
important, but there are also real implications to
essentially shutting down an economy.

March 19

Email from dean of medical education

"Dear Students, I am writing to let you know that one of our
third-year medical students has tested positive for the COVID-19
virus. The student developed symptoms at the end of last week
and is recovering well at home. We are so thankful that our
student is feeling well. We know all of you are following the
guidelines for reducing exposure risk for yourself and others

and are continuing to support each other during these difficult and stressful times."

————

Message received in class GroupMe
Welp, this is significantly awkward. But whoever it is, I hope that you are doing well and recovering. I can't speak for everyone here but let me know if there's anything you need.

————

GRANDPA (76, LIVING IN SINGAPORE)

Everyone is worried about coronavirus. There are some foolish people who prefer to die than take precautions. We have been feeling the stress since December last year. You guys are just feeling it now. But this will last for a while. We are all running for cover. You are in the health industry. You have to work harder than everybody else. Can't escape.

March 20

Hey just fyi I'm headed to O'Hare right now to catch a flight home before the airport shuts down. Stay safe - see y'all whenever. Can somebody pls water my plants while I'm gone?

RUSSELL

Good luck, Sean!!

JASON

Thinking about you! <3

March 24

NEAL

What's up bro? Just checking in seeing how you're doing.

> Hey man school is delayed for now until at least April 6th though assuming it will be later than that. How's the fam?

NEAL

All here in Mason [Ohio]. We're hanging out for the foreseeable future. I'm taking classes online now. My dad still goes into the office, but he's transitioned to Telehealth with his patients. Really hoping he doesn't get called in to do hospital work. Everyone's healthy. Haven't been able to see my grandmother because we're being extra cautious.

What's Sarah up to?

> She came home with me since California is on lockdown.

March 25
Meeting minutes from all-class meeting

- As of this week, there are currently over 40 COVID inpatients being cared for in cohort units
- Physicians and staff are reallocating personnel and resources to handle the increasing number of COVID cases
- Testing remains restricted to inpatients and health care workers with symptoms, due to limited inventory

MS4 Updates

- All remaining required clinical experiences will proceed remotely
- There have been no discussions within leadership regarding the possibility of graduating MS4s early and recruiting them to temporary intern-level work (a la NYU)

MS3 Updates

- On April 6th, students will not return to the wards and will begin remote learning
- Current contingency plans include returning to the wards on April 27th to complete truncated versions of clerkships
    - Regardless of contingency, students will not need to extend their Pritzker education (i.e., take on an extra year) in order to graduate
- Away rotations and sub-Is, on a national level, are still up in the air; we expect significant adjustments in expectations of the residency application process, which at this point are largely unpredictable

MS2 Updates

- Contingency plans are in place in case Prometric closures are prolonged; the exact nature of these plans will depend on the status of MS3 participation on the clinical wards, updates will be forthcoming as soon as next week

MS1 Updates

- Remote learning will begin on April 6th for Cell
  Pathology and Immunology, Microbiology, Clinical
  Skills 1C, and Summer Research; more information
  will be coming from course directors

March 28

Google search

"Hydroxychloroquine"

April 6

Google search

"Boris Johnson"

April 21

JACQUELINE

I was gonna stay in Florida and tell John to
come down but he got corona so I just came
back. I'm glad I'm here now, the student
workforce is actually so much fun.

We got a huge donation of iPads and we've
been configuring them to go on COVID floors in
every patient room so they can talk to their
families and residents can even round on them
from outside the room to conserve PPE.

Shit, is he okay?!? Mt. Sinai is like at the
epicenter.

JACQUELINE

He's 22 days out now and his antibodies are up!
But yeah it's nuts. We finally have COVID
numbers going down. Looks like the peak was
on the 9th. Hopefully there's no second wave
but we shall see.

> I mean Georgia is opening up on the 24th so I
> guess we'll be the guinea pigs...

JACQUELINE

Same with Florida.

sends meme

Entire world: "Stay home"

Florida Man: "No, I don't think I will."

May 25
Google search
"George Floyd"

May 29
Google search
"United States WHO funding withdrawal"

May 31

SARAH

Made it back safely! Already missing y'all.
Thank you for such an amazing stay - can't
properly express how grateful I am.

DAD

Awesome. Also just made it back to the house
after a couple of shopping stops. Seems rather
quiet. Guess I'll go have a drink.

Lots of gunfire and sirens tonight. We're safe.

GEORGIA

There was an alarm going on last night in Atlanta when I was walking Murphy alerting the city about curfew.

———

HUGE protest on 51st. Lootings on 53rd. There are protests everywhere right now. Chi, ATL, NYC. DC is on fire.

June 2

Message received in class GroupMe

Anyone wanna skip their daily workout and clean up some South Side spots with me? I can pick you up, I have bags and brooms.

June 3

Message received in class GroupMe

Dear Colleagues, many of us are angered and saddened by the recent events surrounding the George Floyd, Ahmaud Arbery, and Breonna Taylor cases. As healers, every day we see the effects of racism both overt and systemic in our patients and in some cases feel those effects in our own lives. On June 4, please join us for a peaceful, silent, demonstration as we call attention to the impact that structural racism and social injustice has on our patients, our community and our Country. The intent of this demonstration is a peaceful call to action to promote change. We will not look away while there are whole groups of people in our society who suffer at the hands of structural racism.

Instructions:

- No signs necessary
- Wear work clothes and A MASK
- Stand 6 ft apart in silence while several people read statements
- Approximately 30 minutes - 1 hour

June 26

JINU

How's it been up there? Back to "normal"?

Hospital is at like 75% capacity. Pretty weird being back tho, it's so different than earlier this year. Everybody is wearing masks, we're having socially distant rounds via Zoom most days, also have to take a questionnaire before stepping into the hospital each day to make sure we don't have COVID. Patients aren't allowed to have any family in the room with them either which is pretty heartbreaking.

Had a guy get open heart surgery and his wife was bawling before the surgery because she couldn't say bye in person.

July 24

DAD

Grandaddy has COVID.

GEORGIA

Oh no. How's he doing?

DAD

I think mentally its very heavy on him. Not able to help with your great grandma. Physically very tired and no appetite. Not sure about coughing. He sounded nasally the last two weeks. And weakened voice.

> How did he get it? I thought they were quarantining.

DAD

Don't know. He says he wears gloves and a mask on his few trips out of the house. Grandma's nurse had pneumonia last week.

Carrier?

July 25

GRANDADDY (78, LIVING IN DAHLONEGA, GEORGIA)

When Joey tested positive for COVID, Becky said she didn't have to be tested to know that she had it. That is Barbara [grandmother] - has not been test-verified but she knows she has it.

Our test site is our doctor's office, and they are closed until Monday. She will decide by then if she wants the test. We both slept fairly well last night. She had two or three rounds of sweats like I did the night before. Both have low temps but little to no congestion and only an occasional cough. Lin, Paul, and Bethany have taken over next door for the weekend and the nurse will be back Monday. Hospice is on call if they need them. Conditions next door [Catherine, great-grandmother] are quite low. She did ask to get on the bedside commode during the night and offered some help transferring from and back to the bed. Taking minimal liquids and sometimes a little ice cream to get a pill down.

July 27

GRANDADDY

(Linda's first-hand assessment) Catherine is still hanging in there. Not much change since yesterday. Still not taking food but did accept sips of chicken broth and Boost as well as water. Prayers for mercy, wisdom, and guidance as we move forward.

Barbara feels she has declined a little bit yesterday and today. She is quite sore all over, very little energy or appetite but did seem to sleep a little better last night. She has always had keen hearing but has had difficulty hearing for at least a couple of days - she continues to have a low-grade fever. I feel fairly well today, though I tire rather easily. Have low grade fever this afternoon (99.4) for first time in three days. I slept quite well last night, and I ate a decent brunch around 11:30. Overall I am ok. Just keep the prayers going up.

P.S. Lin and Paul picked the garden this morning, Renee and Bethany snapped the beans, Cathy helped shell peas and Lin, Paul, and Cathy are in the basement kitchen freezing and canning it all. What a blessing. Have a good day.

July 30

GRANDADDY

Catherine is about the same - very restless but not combative, very little sleep. Minimal liquid input - basically what is required to get meds down, minimal liquid output and still nothing solid in or out for a week.

Apparently, she is asking for Barbara this afternoon and Paul is attempting to set up some type of video communication between us. Barbara says she is about like yesterday except could not sleep last night. All vitals are good, hearing is still very poor.

Physically I generally feel almost back to normal, though I don't trust that feeling. All vitals including oxygen level are good with temp remaining a little low (97.7 to 98.3), but I still have night sweats a lot. I can't explain that. I am eating well and lounging lots. Bulletin just came from next door, "Don't be surprised if 'THE CALL' comes tonight."

August 11

Hey man I got an email from the Provost saying medical students should not come tomorrow because of the rioting so unfortunately I won't be in the hospital. Hope to be back Wednesday.

CODY (RESIDENT)

Thanks for the heads up. See you later this week, hopefully.

August 14

GRANDADDY

God declared it "Quittin' Time" for Mrs. Catherine just before 3:00 this morning.

September 10

DAD

Think we're going to the season opener.

Please be careful. There is so much COVID out there.

DAD

Social distance + mask. Stadiums only 25% capacity.

Still 25,000 more than sitting in the living room. For sure positive cases within shouting distance.

DAD

True.

September 26

Google search

"White House Rose Garden Event"

October 2

Wall Street Journal push notification

"A person familiar with Trump's health said there is cause for concern about the president's vital signs, adding that the next 48 hours will be critical."

October 27

Hey just fyi both Sarah and I can't taste or smell our dinner right now so gonna get tested tomorrow. I think more likely than not it's COVID so y'all may want to consider getting tested as well.

DAD

Who cooked? Try something different?

————

Hi, no need to panic yet but I can't really taste my dinner right now. I'm getting tested in the morning and will keep y'all posted. No other symptoms at the moment.

RYAN

Gotcha. I'm also doing voluntary testing tomorrow.

JASON

Thanks for the heads up.

October 28

RYAN

Any result, Sean?

Not yet, assuming I'll hear something tonight.

It's positive.

JASON

Oh shiiiiit.

GENA

Man, that stinks. I'm sorry. Do you feel okay?

Yeah, I feel fine.

October 29

Infectious disease says y'all don't need to get tested since we were outside of 6 feet apart in the home: "greater than 6 feet even without masks is considered no exposure." They say monitor symptoms and get tested if you experience anything but nothing that you need to do at this time.

GENA

Ok! I also called occupational medicine this morning, got a slightly different answer (basically said to quarantine for 5 days and get tested on the 5th day) bc even if we haven't had a direct exposure, we might have had several "cumulative exposures" with just being roommates or something like that.

The waters are probably muddied a bit because really hard to quantify our exposure, but I think overall we'll just generally be careful the next couple days and get tested early next week.

Wow, that's a very different response. It's been surprisingly weird getting answers. The COVID hotline didn't know what contact tracing was. Apologies for the hassle.

GENA

Haha no worries at all! Yeah, I feel like this is definitely not a straightforward situation so hard to give direct answers.

Ok, ID just called me back and backtracked on their previous info. Now it's more consistent with what they told you, Gena, that y'all should get tested as early as tomorrow. Apparently MyChart has easy scheduling.

October 30

Google search

"Should I take prophylactic aspirin for COVID?"

November 2

Email from dean of medical education

"Dear Pritzker School of Medicine Students, we are, of course, protecting the privacy of our students, but we did want to share with the community that the medical school has recorded a very small number of positive cases of COVID-19 within our student body. We would like to reassure the general student body that active contact tracing has been undertaken, and those who have been in contact with these students would already know of their potential exposure."

———

RYAN

How are you guys doing over at Ellis? Still feeling okay?

Getting better each day. Everybody over here tested negative, so things are looking up.

November 3
Google search
"538 election tracker"

November 4
Google search
"538 election tracker"

November 5
Google search
"538 election tracker"

November 6
Google search
"538 election tracker"

November 7
Google search
"538 election tracker"

December 11
Google search
"Pfizer vaccine"

December 18
Google search
"Moderna vaccine"

January 6
Google search
"US Capitol attack"

January 16

GRANDADDY

Thought I would let you know that I have just taken my first COVID vaccine shot and am writing this as I wait for 15 minutes to see if I have any reactions.

It was the Pfizer vaccine. I called the Lumpkin County health department phone number yesterday to make a reservation and was told that they had no more vaccines available, but they would check White County. The receptionist came back after checking and said that White and Dawson Counties had none, but Hall County had some if I wanted to go there. I had my calendar in hand turned to March, hoping to get an appointment by then. But he said, "I can give you an appointment at 9:15 tomorrow if you want it." In shock that I could get an appointment in an adjoining county immediately when Lumpkin and two other neighboring counties had none, I told him I would take the appointment, and here I am.

I had the shot 20 minutes ago and no negative reactions. I am grateful.

March 14

Email from The New York Times

"Your Weekend Briefing: One year in a pandemic. A special edition looking at a year of living in disruption and pain."

March 17

Email from dean of medical education

"Dear Pritzker Community, we are sharing the statement which circulated earlier today from the Department of Medicine Diversity Committee regarding recent violence against Asian-

Americans in our country. We at the Pritzker School of Medicine strongly endorse this statement and join in condemning in the strongest terms this violence and prejudice. We too stand together with our Asian-American faculty, house staff, students, staff, patients, and communities in condemning acts of discrimination and hatred."

April 20
Email from the American Medical Association
"AMA Morning Rounds: All Americans 16 and older now eligible for COVID-19 vaccines"

April 25

> ROB
>
> First vaccine scheduled. LFG.
>
> Loved "First vaccine scheduled. LFG."

15

A DIFFERENT KIND OF LOVE

I don't understand why people insist on pitting concepts of evolution and creation against each other. Why can't they see that spiritualism and science are one? That bodies evolve and souls evolve and the universe is a fluid package that marries them both in a wonderful package called a human being. What's wrong with that idea?

—Garth Stein, *The Art of Racing in the Rain*

I LIVED MOST of my childhood in Suwanee, Georgia. In the heart of the Bible Belt, I was raised in a Southern Baptist family. By nature of this upbringing, more often than not, on Sunday mornings, I went to church with my mom, dad, and older sister. Church began promptly at 11:00 a.m. and lasted an hour. Afterward, we would stop by the neighborhood Applebee's on the way home, or if we were in a rush to a ballgame or cheerleading competition, the Panda Express on State Route 141.

I never did like going to the youth service. Maybe it was because the music consisted of an acoustic guitar playing the same four songs on a loop, or maybe it was that the youth pastor's personality perfectly matched those "*youth pastor voice*" memes circulating on Twitter ("Do you understand why we stan Jesus? Well, here's the tea." "You know who else lived Among Us? Our Lord and Savior Jesus Christ." "Guess what other royal family member left his throne for love?"). Whatever the reason, I tended to avoid the services geared toward kids my own age, and as a result, I tagged along with my parents to the adult sermon. There, I would find myself surrounded by men with thinning hair and women with handbags full of hard candy.

In the pulpit, most Sundays after the organ ceased playing, the preacher would stand behind a podium with a wireless mic fastened to his ear, discussing topics that went far over my head. The divine relationship of the Trinity. The concept of eschatology. The parable of The Prodigal Son. Still, every now and again, the scripture would offer a nugget of wisdom that resonated deep within my still-developing mind. On one particular occasion, the topic was love. The preacher began his argument with its definition. More precisely, he explained how, in the Bible, there existed several distinct types. Because the New Testament was originally written in Greek, each form of love was easily discernable, as they were associated with their own discrete words: storge, philias, eros, and agape.

As a kid, I had not yet experienced the depths of these loves in any fashion (aside from within my immediate family), but I wanted to, and I filed away their essences for a later date. Had I been asked then, I would have found relief at my good fortune of witnessing the richest of each as they played out before me in the individuals I would later meet on the wards, in their stories, in their smallest of actions performed in caring for one another.

Each scene, I know now, would consistently bring me back to the church where I grew up in Suwanee, Georgia, surrounded by men in plaid suits and women with large hats.

Storge love, the preacher said, was a familial love. It was love of kin. It was affectionate. It was warm. At the start of my neurology rotation, I was assigned to the stroke service, where I saw in every patient the face of hardship. Each had thrown a clot into an important brain structure—the middle cerebral artery, the vessels of the internal capsule, the pons—the details of which no longer mattered to the patients because the outcome remained a catastrophic loss of function, such as an inability to form words, loss of motor function, or hemineglect. From my years in undergrad studying neuroplasticity through a micro-scope, I knew more than most that restoration of brain function, if at all, would happen slowly over the course of days to weeks to months.

On this rotation, I took care of a patient who had suffered a massive left-sided stroke. By the time he made it up to the ninth floor of the Center for Care and Discovery, he was partially para-lyzed, unable to talk, and had an impaired cough reflex. He had frequent oral secretions pooling in his throat, which required the use of a tube hooked up to wall suction in order to prevent aspiration of his own saliva. Because he could not eat, and in spite of his copious secretions, his constant state of dehydration meant his mouth often felt dry. On rounds, he would ask me, through his daughter, to fetch him ice chips to quench his thirst.

In the mornings when I stopped by, I found myself struck by the way his daughter cared for him. No matter the time of day, she could be found sitting on the vinyl couch below the window, scribbling notes in the three-ring binder which she used to track his updates. What I admired most in this relationship was how, in a few short days, she had learned an entirely new language. The twitch of her dad's mouth meant he wanted ice chips. The flinch of his neck muscles meant suction was requested. A long blink meant that he was uncomfortable and desired repositioning. A garbled monosyllable meant that he wanted his mouth wiped. She heeded these calls almost subconsciously, lifting his head to adjust his pillow in the middle of informing me of how her father's speech therapy session went earlier in the day, reaching for a suction tube in between pauses as if to say, "I am with you, we are here together. Do not worry." Her compassion was pure, the kind only existing between parent and child.

Philias love, the preacher told me, was brotherly, fraternal, bound by friendship. Later, on the same clerkship, I cared for an elderly immigrant from mainland China who was experiencing a strange constellation of symptoms. He was a squatty man with wispy black hair which fell just north of his bushy brows. He brought with him to the hospital a tattered collared shirt, beige in color with several navy stripes spaced at arbitrary intervals, which, for some reason, he preferred to wear instead of the gown we had provided him. He had a kind demeanor and eyes that made me feel appreciated. Since he only spoke Cantonese, I communicated with him through a "language line," a translation service available to patients through the telephones in their rooms. The process for securing the translation service was laborious and time intensive, and so, instead of subjecting ourselves to the discordant tones of on-hold music each day, we settled on a new routine. My patient's most frequent visitor, who I would come to learn was his lifelong friend, became our go-between.

Other than appreciating his assistance with the initial interview, I found his friend to be abrasive. He was often jovial with the patient when I entered the room, but held his tongue in our encounters, speaking up only to challenge my requests for a lumbar puncture or interject with questions from an unidentified Chinese physician whom he conferenced in from back home. He asked brooding questions and did not seem satisfied by my inability to provide answers about the then mystery of the patient's condition. It was from him that I learned that the patient's main complaint was blurry vision. Upon further inspection, I noticed that the patient was unable to keep his eyes open for long, specifically struggling to look up toward the ceiling. He nearly toppled over when I requested that he stand, and once upright, he walked with a shuffling gait.

We started with a shotgun diagnostic approach, testing for a variety of neurological conditions which might have been to blame: myasthenia gravis, multiple sclerosis, neurosyphilis, paraneoplastic disease, progressive supranuclear palsy. After several rounds of tests, we discovered that the patient had been suffering from a disease known as Miller Fischer syndrome, a rare autoimmune disorder thought to be caused by an inflammatory reaction to a resolved viral infection. He was started on intravenous immunoglobulin, IVIG for short, in order to sequester the antibodies responsible for his condition.

I noticed the friend's disposition notably shift when I was finally able to describe to him our assessment and treatment plan. It seemed to me that the stress had melted off his body before my eyes, revealing an entirely different person underneath. He began smiling, he shook my hand, and he finally felt comfortable enough to leave the room when I was speaking with the patient. I knew then that my original read of contempt on his behalf was coming from a place of genuine concern, of care, of love between friends.

Eros love, in contrast, was romantic love. It was the kind of love felt for a partner: physical, sexual, and erotic. On the night shift of my general surgery rotation, I spent the hours from midnight to two in the morning conducting "post-op" checks on patients who had just undergone surgery. The goal of these visits was to make sure that, in the period immediately following an operation, a patient's vital signs remained stable, and they were not experiencing an acute clinical decline as a result of a new complication (heart attack, internal bleeding, altered mental status, etc.). On these rounds, I found most patients asleep when I knocked on their doors. I would usually wake them gently to press on their bellies and ask if they had passed any stool or gas, an encouraging sign of bowel motility. I would ask about any fevers or chills, chest pain, or shortness of breath. Assuming all was well, I would then tell them that the day team would come and check on them in the morning before shutting the door on my way out.

One night, as I approached a patient room in the short stay area of the hospital, I noticed the fluorescent glow of blue light poking through the crack in the bottom of the door. The rooms in the short stay area were arranged such that behind the door was a floor-to-ceiling drape that slid along a railing like a shower curtain. When pulled taut, a passerby from the hallway would not be able to see the patient through the window of the door. This was how I found many rooms, and I thought nothing more of this. Anyway, I had more patients to see.

I knocked twice then entered. As the door swung open, I heard a rustle from the other side as I reached out in the shadows to grab the curtain. The metallic scraping of ball bearings caterwauled as it drew open, slowly exposing the bed in which my patient was lying. I first noticed the gown on the floor, then two eyes reflecting back at me from the head of the bed, before finally recognizing a mass roughly the size of another human body hiding under the sheets. In a situation like this, there was nothing more to say other than to do my job: "I am so sorry, have you had any bowel movements since the operation?"

From these interactions and beautiful accidents, I had seen storge, philias, and even eros on the wards. Through them, I recognized how each was a manifestation of love's unique forms. At the same time, I was also surprised to have noticed them in this setting. I suppose I should not have been, for rarely elsewhere were these snapshots of love so prominently broadcast for display. This appeared to be the case, by my observation, because hospital patients are stripped of the locks on their doors and the shirts on their backs so that we can consistently see, behind all layers of privacy, heartbreakingly precious human interactions through tiny glimpses of who they were, who they are, who they will be.

This is an unintended consequence of medicine for which I hold little affection, but in each instance, I do feel honored to have been able to watch all of these representations of a kind of intimacy so unlike what I'd observed in the world outside the white walls of Mitchell Hospital. Witnessing a wordless conversation shared between a father and a daughter, between two friends, between lovers, I was awestruck. If a movie were made of these moments, I would see myself watching the characters enact the scene before me. I know my eyes would dart around, shying away from the action at hand and looking anywhere else around the room, almost embarrassed—not for the patients and their loved ones but for myself having been a part of this. I would recognize that I was an intruder in these moments, watching the personification of wedding vows, "in sickness and in health," seeing the worst parts of their care but the best parts of their love: storge, philias, eros in the flesh.

The final form of love also grew out of medicine, but it was one that could not be seen in others and had to be experienced. The preacher told me that agape love was perfect, infinite, absolute.

I met Sarah on the first night of her Second Look Weekend during the spring of my first year in medical school. She approached me at a party and asked if I was an incoming student. I made a dumb quip about how I was not, and we went our separate ways. By the end of the second night, we had spent an hour talking to one another, and in that time, I learned about the other schools she was considering, her childhood growing up in San Diego with two brothers, and her affinity for horrible puns. By the end of the third night, we had our first kiss. After the weekend was over, I asked for her number and we texted throughout the summer.

We dated into the fall of my MS2 year, and in September, on my birthday, she handed me a note referencing *The Fault in Our Stars* along with her own improvisation tacked on at the end:

> *John Green, an author I was obsessed with in high*
> *school, once described falling in love as being akin*
> *to falling asleep—slowly and then all at once. I*
> *feel like this is only accurate in my case if I use the*
> *way you fall asleep—rapidly, and in massive*
> *bursts that seem almost impossible.*

Sarah's experience largely mirrored mine. The first few months of dating, we somersaulted, head over heels. When she moved to Chicago, we went on dates to sushi dinners, to White Sox games, to arboretums. On each, we talked about our families and our lives before starting medical school, what we valued and who we aspired to become. We traveled to Phoenix and Nashville and San Francisco for research conferences and explored the cities together in between lectures. I took her as my date to our medical school formal. She met my best friends. In all of these nights in and nights out, we were together. Life got busier with school, but she was my constant.

On our first Valentine's Day a little less than a year after we met, I finally said those three words. Things accelerated from there. For winter break, I took Sarah to spend time with my parents. During this stay, I had arranged a brief excursion to Savannah, Georgia. We drove down there for the weekend, and on that Friday, I had planned a walking tour of the city. We grabbed lunch at one of the restaurants on River Street, after which we stopped by the City Market before ambling over to Chippewa Square and then to the Mercer House. We had plans to finish on the south side of town before calling it an afternoon, but by the time we arrived at the Cathedral Basilica of St. John the Baptist, the bottom fell out of the sky. We took shelter there for a few minutes to look at the radar, which showed no signs of the rain relenting, before deciding to continue our heroes' quest onward in the tempest. I picked her up on my back and carried her over puddles on our journey to the last stop, the fountain at Forsyth Park.

Once there, we paused to take in the scene, and what a scene it was. Above our heads, our umbrella mercifully held strong, refusing to yield to the battering of the downpour. Each raindrop coalesced into larger streams atop this polyester canopy, cascading over the edge at an impressive speed before splashing to the ground around our ankles. Through the waterfall, we could see the stone path we had used to get here littered with puddles, glistening with each entropic force, lined on either side of the path by century-old live oaks draped delicately in Spanish moss. In the darkness of the storm, at the end of the walkway, a statue stood in the middle of the fountain, glowing a radiant white. It sustained its own cyclical ejection of water in an audacious protest as if unimpressed by the fervor of the storm. We stood here for quite some time, holding onto each other, and in that moment, this was the world we inhabited. Nobody dared impose. I felt so at home.

When the pandemic hit and brought our world to a screeching halt, Sarah and I spent nearly three months back with my parents in the north Georgia mountains. We had been sent home in the name of student safety, and in place of rotations, we picked up several classes and new research deadlines, but for the most part, we just lived together, experiencing the first glimmer of our futures, talking about adopting cats and having kids and moving in together for real. Our favorite place to have these conversations was down by a small pond at the edge of my parents' property, a place we considered a little piece of paradise. The pond was fed by dozens of natural mountain springs which merged into a babbling brook. Down the mountain it tumbled onto a flat piece of land where the previous owner had created a dam. Here, he had populated the pond with a few goldfish which over the years had reproduced to establish a thriving community among the bullfrogs, snapping turtles, and water spiders. We enjoyed our near daily walks here as the world crumbled around us, and from the security of this venue, we watched the seasons change. We experienced the barren trees of winter, where a shout would echo unimpeded throughout the valley. We saw springtime, when the winds would carry white blooms through the air like a snowstorm in April. We were there for summer, when we would see deer and wild turkey and black bears wander the woods in search of food. Often during these talks, the sun would set in the western sky, behind the blue ridges made up of green needles. It was perfection.

When the virus was somewhat better understood, we eventually went back to school, me to finish up my final year and Sarah to complete her third. Because the pandemic had wreaked havoc on her schedule, she had an eight-week period after the conclusion of her clerkships during which she needed to take both parts one and two of the boards. Since we'd had an enjoyable time at my parents' home in Ellijay, she chose to spend her study block in May and June there with them. As I geared up for graduation, I had the luxury of time and elected to spend it with them as well.

As we had in quarantine, in the evenings, we would often take walks to the pond, Sarah lugging a bucket of fish food and me a sand wedge and a handful of golf balls. She would shovel the pebbles into the expectant mouths circling in the depths below while I would tinker around with beat up Maxfli Noodles, picking pitch shots cleanly off the mossy carpet and sending projectiles into the hillside back toward the house.

One afternoon, following a day full of studying, we went on the walk that had become so dear to us. It was a classic late spring day in the mountains of North Georgia. The air was fresh and the water calm, reflecting back the undersides of leaves and the puffy white clouds blowing overhead. When we arrived, I handed Sarah, for her editorial review, the draft of a new chapter I had written. She had grown accustomed to this routine over the past couple years. She told me that she appreciated

reading these musings, and I valued the feedback she provided
—what she thought worked and what didn't, which jokes might
have landed and which fell flat. The entire time she read, I
eagerly waited for her to finish, as I always did. When she finally
reached the end, it read:

> *Agape is the highest form of love. It is reverent. It is
> unconditional. It is what I feel for you. Sarah, will
> you marry me?*

MS4

16

MONGOOSE

For me, becoming isn't about arriving somewhere or achieving a certain aim. I see it instead as forward motion, a means of evolving, a way to reach continuously toward a better self. The journey doesn't end.

—Michelle Obama, *Becoming*

WITH THE END of third year came the end of many wonderful things. I had met individuals who had forever shaped my outlook on medicine and life, and I had shared experiences with classmates which brought us closer together as caretakers and as humans.

Thankfully, with the end of third year came the end of many frustrating things as well. It was the end of spending countless hours in the hospital investing energy in fields I did not necessarily envision myself ever entering. It was the end of feeling the need to feign enthusiasm for the daily annoyances that accompanied being at the bottom of the totem pole. It was the end of being scrutinized over the most ridiculous and minute of details, many of which were irrelevant to patient care.[i]

For all the good and the bad, MS3 did serve a greater purpose. By the end of the year, after gaining exposure to a variety of medical disciplines, we were expected to ultimately decide on a specialty to which we would apply. Out of this necessity, on each rotation, we pondered whether or not we found the material interesting, working with the patient population rewarding, and the lifestyle sustainable. We additionally considered how we might fit into each field's culture and whether the stereotypes we had heard about since matriculating into medical school held any substance. Were anesthesiologists all about the ABCs (Airway, Breathing, Coffee Breaks)? Did general surgeons really throw instruments across the operating room when they were mad? Was it possible that dermatologists were passionate about skin before crushing Step 1? Could I find an extroverted radiologist, a urologist without a sense of humor, or a neurosurgeon without a god complex? And what did pediatricians eat in the morning to make them so pleasant?

After a clinical year spent dabbling in a number of different specialties, I had chosen to apply into orthopedic surgery. I offi-

---

[i]   Grades during third year essentially amount to a letter system: Honors (A), High Pass (B), Pass (C), Fail (F). On each rotation, attendings and residents subjectively evaluate students based on their judgment of a student's knowledge of practice, data gathering skills, communication of data, clinical reasoning, management, interpersonal communication skills, professionalism, procedural skills, teamwork, health promotion and prevention, and potential as a resident in each discipline. These grades, unlike the pass-fail grading structure of the first two years, function to rank students against their peers, and they are ultimately used by residency programs for job placement in the fourth year.

came to this conclusion after spending two weeks rotating with the department during third year, though admittedly, the groundwork had been laid years prior with several research projects and shadowing opportunities. Still, throughout the elective, I considered what it was about the field that I found appealing, and on the final day of the rotation, I scribbled the first few sentences of what would ultimately comprise part of my personal statement:

> *It's interesting being a medical student with a long-term condition. Every time I step into the doctor's office, not in the seat I will one day occupy but through the lens of a patient, I find myself as both student and teacher. The more I occupy this space the more I realize I will never fully escape this identity. At each appointment I'll lie back as my doctor palpates and auscultates the way she always does. I'll cling to her every word and with each visit gain insight into the kind of doctor I want to be. In a sense this is both terrifying and liberating, and maybe it's out of this fear or rebelliousness that I first fell in love with orthopedics - because the field represented the exact opposite of the condition with which I am afflicted. It can cure, it offers immediacy and longevity, and it is mentally and physically stimulating.*

I think this sentiment still holds true years after these words were written. I've seen patients who virtually walk out of total knee replacements, kids with scoliosis who stand two inches taller after a spine fusion, and even my own dad with a repaired biceps tendon FaceTiming me after a day of chainsawing trees in the backyard. It was also true that being forced to grapple with a chronic condition framed what I sought from a career. After my diagnosis, I knew I no longer had a choice in how I managed my disease. I was told that I needed to take medication and I did, and like nearly all medications, it was not curative. Naturally, the lack of finality irritated me, and when the time came to decide what to do with my life, I thought it would be infinitely gratifying to go to work and fix people in ways that only surgery could. As a surgeon, I would be the one putting broken bones back together, replacing failing joints, and helping people dance again. I don't know if I would have stumbled into orthopedics had I not been pushed in this direction, but here I was.

After this decision, the remainder of fourth year was largely build-your-own. Broadly speaking, it included a sub-internship (a monthlong audition in the chosen specialty at one's home institution), one to three away rotations (monthlong auditions in the chosen specialty at outside institutions), teaching assistant positions for first- and second-year courses, and various other nonclinical electives tailored toward specific interests, such as Money Management for the Young Physician or Genetics. Regardless of specialty selection, universally, a medical student's responsibilities increased in the promotion from MS3 to MS4. At this point in our medical school careers, as a sub-intern or away rotator, it was suddenly expected that we would carry a higher patient load, place orders in the chart, and prepare the list in the mornings for the intern on service. Our presentations on rounds were also assumed to be polished and our differentials crisp. Because orthopedic surgery was so subspecialized, however, nowhere in medical school did we receive any formal teaching in this subject matter. As a result, when I started my sub-intern-ship, I was advised by former students to sit back and observe for the first few days, to carefully take mental notes of things like each attending's preferred operative setup or the materials gathered from the supply closet prior to splinting a fracture. Once I had a better idea of what was going on, I could jump into the action.

I woke up on the first day of the rotation eager to finally start learning the material I would need to know to practice in this discipline. I walked into the trauma operating room and introduced myself to the team, and I looked on, excited to help as instructed, as the residents buzzed around grabbing bone foam and sticky tape.

About thirty seconds after wheeling the patient into the OR, the attending turned toward me. "What are you doing?" he demanded. "In the OR, I have a job." He pointed at the resident as he continued, "He has a job. You have a job. Let's get moving —you can't just stand there."

That set the tone for what would be an intense month. I had ordered a fracture handbook off Amazon and anatomy flash-cards, and I studied during every bit of downtime I had between surgeries. No matter how much I studied, though, in the OR, I would field questions about operative intervals, fracture classifications, and surgical indications to which I did not know the answers. In the evenings, I would attend lectures and wonder how my co-students knew what a Velpeau view of the shoulder was or that a primary anterior cruciate ligament (ACL) repair— instead of a reconstruction—was even an option. At the end of each day full of questioning and correcting, I could not help but feel defeated and generally fatigued from my own idiocy, but perhaps more tiring was the constant need to put myself in a position exposing my lack of understanding. In order to be taught, I had to admit that I did not know. To get it right the next time, I had to fail the first time. This was something that I have never enjoyed.

In the second grade, Mrs. Anthony asked the class who made the first American flag. She projected an image on the board with red and white stripes and thirteen stars in the top left corner oriented in a big circle. I threw my hand into the air and stared at her. She scanned the room, and when our eyes locked, she sighed before gesturing in my direction. I opened my mouth and attempted to say "Betsy Ross," but instead what accidentally squeaked out was the name "Betty Crocker." My face turned bright red, and I hid my shame in the crease of my elbow. Everybody laughed.

In the seventh grade, most of my friends started playing first-person-shooter video games like Call of Duty and Halo. I thought it sounded fun and wanted to play against them online, so for Christmas that year, I asked my parents for an Xbox 360. After much pleading, they finally caved. When it arrived a few months later, I smiled to myself as I created the gamertag "PirkleNurple" and shortly thereafter logged into Xbox Live for the first time.

I knew early on that I was the worst of the group. Since I had joined months after everyone had started playing, they had all already memorized the maps and knew which sections to avoid; meanwhile, I aimlessly wandered into live claymores and sniper traps, pulling the team down with me along the way. In most of these games, after a character died, there would be a brief, live camera feed hovering over the scene while a player waited to respawn. During these times after I had been slain, more often than not, I would see my friends running over from across the screen to virtually teabag my corpse as they made fun of how high-pitched my voice was over my wireless headset mic. When I went to a friend's birthday party later that year, everybody wanted to play Call of Duty. I sat and watched the whole time.

The theme continued into college. Shortly after graduation, I had a couple months to kill before the start of medical school. At the time, I had an interest in the world of business and figured, before starting a career in medicine, that it could be fun to dabble in consulting. I attended a few information sessions held on campus that spring and learned that certain firms seemed to appreciate having MDs on board. I submitted applications to a handful of potential summer internships at McKinsey, Bain, and the Boston Consulting Group (BCG) and waited. Three weeks later, I received an email from one of the companies informing me of my upcoming "case interview."

As a premed major, I had no idea what this meant, but when I asked a friend, she panicked for me. I learned very quickly that the case interview, while niche to consulting, was nearly universally used. Acing one would apparently require a strong background in economics, including real-time interpretations of charts and graphs, a heavy dose of mental math, and a series of well-approximated assumptions (e.g., population of the US, success rates of pharmaceutical drug discovery, number of patients insured through private and public means).

A medical consulting interviewer might pose a scenario such as this: "Company A, which makes small molecule drugs like aspirin, is looking to acquire Company B, specializing in biologic drugs that target the immune response." They would then ask a series of wide-ranging questions which the interviewee must systematically approach to extract the required information, such as: "How big is this new market?" or

"What are the margins on Drug B?" In the end, once the interviewee has attempted to walk through their thought process, the interviewer would likely circle back to the original question and ask for a formal recommendation.

Since these interviews were extremely nuanced, candidates would spend months preparing for their first one. I had six days.

As the day neared, I felt an unmistakable sense of impending doom. I had watched a series of YouTube videos and asked my friend to conduct a mock interview, both of which only served to highlight my deficiencies and heighten my anxiety. I heavily considered dropping the interview but decided to see it through because I felt that, even in the worst-case scenario, it would be a good opportunity for personal development. When the interview came, I was so nervous that I lost the ability to do all mental math. I did not get the job.

I still think back in horror at these mistakes because they were so emotionally vexing. Unfortunately for me, these were the memories that came rushing into my psyche during my sub-internship every time I forced myself into a position where failing was the most likely outcome: asking stupid questions during journal club; committing to diagnoses in clinic that were way off base; making flimsy splints knowing, as I was wrapping it, that the resident would have to redo it immediately after me. In all of this, I looked at the interns and saw an impossible amount of distance between where I was and where I needed to be. I knew I had less than a year to get there and thought that I would never be able to bridge the gap.

———

When I was five years old, I had a red Mongoose mountain bike. I picked it out at Walmart because I thought the badger-like-creature running down the side looked cool (I later learned, in a shocking turn of events, that the logo was, in fact, a mongoose). The bike came with thick rubber tires, a turtle shell helmet, and two training wheels attached at the back. Most days after school, I could be found riding this bike with my first gang, Trevor on his own Mongoose and Dylan from a few doors down on a Razr scooter.

One day, my dad took a screwdriver to the back wheel and asked me to meet him outside. I protested for a bit before walking the bike down the slope of my driveway and into the cul-de-sac. There, he scooped me up, placed me atop the seat, and flanked my hands with his on either side of the handlebars. We went around in circles like this for some time, my legs churning us forward and his arms steadying us upright. A dozen revolutions later, he moved his hands to the back of my seat and promised, in doing so, that he would not let go. Still, I looked back at regular intervals to ensure he had not broken our agreement, each time comforted by his continued presence, jogging behind me as I wobbled ahead under my own direction. I'm not quite sure when, but in one of those loops he let go.

Our mentors can never really be sure, when we are pushed out of the nest, if we will fly or flail, sink or swim, stay upright or find ourselves with scraped knees in the neighbor's bushes. They can only make general assumptions based on our past performance or where previous mentees were at a similar time in their training. Regardless of the outcome, I am not convinced any of it matters. Whether we succeed on the first try is but a blip on a journey toward a fixed endpoint. Our mentors know that, at some point along the way, we will eventually fall, we will eventually fail, and we will eventually make mistakes. They know this because they themselves were once the ones falling, and they themselves were once the ones who were forced to get back up.

Success and failure are so intimately intertwined. To be able to do one, we have to be able to do the other. In medicine, learning happens by "seeing one, doing one, then teaching one," and the most important aspect of this cycle happens when we make that leap from seeing to doing. Self-improvement happens in those moments of struggle, where we must be willing to not look back and check if there is a hand steadying us upright. We must lean into the fear and uncertainty and see where they take us, to be willing to fall and fall hard, so long as we get back up afterward and try again. The tough part of this passage is that the points of inflection are never really a choice. We don't get to pick to fail this time and succeed the next, and it is equally difficult to know if and how we are growing until looking back in retrospect.

In the blink of an eye, the sub-internship was over. In the time spent between this rotation and the submission of residency applications, I had signed up to be a teaching assistant for four MSIs working their way through the clinical skills curriculum. In this role, every other week for a semester, I would walk over to the old student lounge to field questions from them about how to not blow out a patient's eardrum when inserting an otoscope or the difference between the "lub" and the "dub" of each heart sound. They would apologize profusely for how seemingly simplistic their questions were, and in response, I would laugh and tell them about how when I first received my stethoscope, I didn't even know which direction the earpieces faced.

Later that semester, I received a call from a family friend complaining about pain in his hand. I took a quick history and made the diagnosis of trigger finger before recommending a corticosteroid injection and hanging up the phone. I got a text a week later letting me know that he had received his injection and it had resolved his symptoms.

I will never know the exact moment when my dad let go, but I will always know the feeling of turning back and realizing he was no longer holding on. Every progression is stepwise— whether we're learning to ride a bike or to become a doctor. At each transition point, there is no real change in ability from one day to the next, and graduated responsibility always seems to come in tranches. At different points in time, we go from MS3s to MS4s, from sub-interns to interns, from residents to attendings. The training wheels come off, the parent figure goes inside, and we are left on our own, biking around in circles until our dinner is ready.

17

THE MATCH

We don't need a legacy
We don't need money
If I could grant you peace of mind
If you could let me inside your heart
Oh, let me be a part of the narrative
In the story they will write someday
Let this moment be the first chapter
Where you decide to stay
And I could be enough
And we could be enough
That would be enough

—Lin-Manuel Miranda and Phillipa Soo, "That Would Be Enough"

THE FIRST RESIDENCY PROGRAM, as we know it, was formally established in 1889 by Dr. William Osler at Johns Hopkins

University. Since its inception, and enduring more than a half a century later, this initial process of hiring new interns created an environment of increasing chaos. You can imagine how the parties involved—medical students and hospital systems, each with opposing stakes at play—contributed uniquely to the absurdity.

In the early days, a hospital system competed against hundreds of others to recruit the best crop of trainees. As such, hospitals benefited from extending offers to qualified candidates as early as possibly identified, before another could poach top talent. Students, rather, in an ideal scenario, sought to train at a program that most aligned with their priorities, whether that be the institution with the most prestigious pedigree, the most robust facilities, or the best location, with proximity to family, friends, or the trappings of a large metropolitan area. They, therefore, stood to benefit from fielding multiple offers and holding onto them until the last minute, scrutinizing the pros and cons of each opportunity, and when the time came, selecting the program that was the right fit. Largely due to the power held over trainees as the party offering the job, hospitals began slowly soliciting prospective applications earlier and earlier each successive year. By the 1940s, programs were offering medical students internship positions as early as their junior year in medical school, nearly two years prior to the position's start date.

This practice itself was not necessarily detrimental to a student's will. For instance, I would have been hard pressed to find any of my colleagues complaining about having a job years before graduation. To make this more chaotic, though, most of the offers from hospitals were "exploding," and it was not unheard of for the offer to expire within the week of the initial contact. The hospital system's logic behind this approach held that, if they were unable to succeed with their first pick, another competing hospital might be calling, in real time, their next best applicant(s). By the time their first pick rejected them, it might then be far too late to find an eligible replacement. As a student receiving this call, one would be faced with a challenging decision: to accept the exploding offer or decline it and assume the risk of waiting for a call from a different (potentially better) institution that might or might not ever come. It often led students to prematurely accept positions at less desirable institutions to avoid the risk of not finding a job entirely.

Clearly, this was a problem. In fact, it was one first identified back in the 1920s, when this whole residency application process was cementing itself in the fabric of the American healthcare system. In an open letter to the Association of American Medical Colleges (AAMC), then-dean of the Columbia College of Physicians and Surgeons Dr. William Darrach advocated for increasing selflessness in hospital systems' hiring practices. Dr. Darrach backed his words with action, vowing in 1927 that, the same year, New York Presbyterian would delay the hiring of interns until after the start of students' fourth year in medical school. By establishing a later hiring date, Dr. Darrach hoped to kickstart a more collaborative environment among hospital systems, effectively alleviating stress on both ends. Of course, this policy would require widespread adoption and would collapse in any cycle where just a single bad player gamed the system by offering jobs early to exceptional candidates and subsequently having their pick of the lot. This scenario describes the tragedy of the commons, and unsurprisingly, this was what happened for over two decades after Dr. Darrach's initial warning.

Beginning around 1945 and leading into the next decade, however, attempts to resolve the practice of early offers gained momentum, with medical schools agreeing to a "Cooperative Plan" prohibiting the release of student information (i.e., transcripts, class rank) until a universally agreed-upon date in students' fourth year. Hospitals responded by shortening the timeline before an offer exploded. In the year the Cooperative Plan was founded, internship offers remained open for a minimum of ten days. During this time, students would be free to field calls and ruminate over the decision with their loved ones. Nevertheless, just four years later, a deadline of twelve hours was rejected by the American Hospital Association (AHA) as being too *long*. It was also increasingly more commonplace for a residency program to offer a job via telegram and then call the applicant immediately afterward, requesting an answer by the end of the conversation. The Cooperative Plan had failed.

In 1950, F.J. Mullin proposed a solution called the Centralized Match. The match would be based on an algorithm which tabulated applicant and hospital rank lists, and it was theoretically coded to "maximize satisfaction" on both sides of the aisle by attempting to pair an applicant with their first, then second, then third (and so on) hospital choice, provided the hospital(s) wanted to hire the student as well.

To demonstrate this point, if I sought to train at hospitals in California, New York, and Texas in that order, I would list the hospitals consecutively on my rank list. Based on my preferences, the algorithm would attempt to match me at my first choice. If the hospital in California ranked me high enough to match, I would match there. Easy. However, if the hospital in California did not like me and ranked me further down on their list, other more-qualified students would match there and fill their available positions for hire, and the algorithm would then attempt to match me at my second choice: New York. If the hospital in New York ranked me highly, then I would match there, but if not, the algorithm would try again and attempt to match me in Texas. If the hospital in Texas ranked me highly, then I would match at my third choice. If they did not rank me highly, and I had no more hospitals on my rank list, I would go unmatched.

This process went on for several decades until Kevin Williams, then a fourth-year medical student at Johns Hopkins University, recognized a fundamental problem with the match algorithm: there was more than one solution. In his 1981 paper published in the *New England Journal of Medicine*, he and several classmates used existing mathematics and economics literature to describe how maximizing satisfaction between applicants and hospitals could work in multiple directions, and the orientation of the algorithm determined who was proposing to whom. He realized that the National Resident Matching Program (NRMP) was oriented such that it was program favoring, allowing the hospitals to have their first choice as opposed to the applicants. For the next twenty years, Dr. Williams continued to advocate on behalf of students until his ideas finally attained widespread traction in his 1995 paper on algorithmic bias. In response, the NRMP conceded and hired mathematicians who ultimately confirmed Dr. Williams' claims and adjusted the code of the match algorithm to be "applicant favoring."

There have been many other minor adjustments to the code as the years have passed to account for an increasing number of couples applying or for those applying into more than one specialty, but for simplicity's sake, since 1952, the backbone of the match has been based on this principle of the "stable marriage," an idea which would go on to win Drs. Lloyd Shapley and Alvin Roth the Nobel Memorial Prize in Economic Sciences in 2012.

With this background in mind, the present-day residency application officially opens in August of the fourth year. A website called the Electronic Residency Application Service (ERAS) houses each student's information in a database, much like the Common Application for applying to college or the American Medical College Application Service (AMCAS) for medical school. Like prior application cycles, each medical student uploads their grades and board scores, their awards and research engagements, and details of their community and institutional service. They then submit a personal statement professing their love for their chosen specialty, and they round out the package with three to five letters of recommendation.

Once all of this has been accomplished, they apply to anywhere between fifteen and 120 different programs, a number varying dramatically by specialty. For traditionally less competitive specialties (which experience higher match rates) like family medicine, pathology, neurology, and internal medicine, an applicant can typically feel comfortable finding a match applying to fewer (15–30) programs. Conversely, for more competitive surgical subspecialities (which experience lower match rates) like otolaryngology, thoracic surgery, neurosurgery, plastic surgery, and orthopedic surgery, a broader application spread is recommended. As of this writing, each program charges a fixed amount of money to submit an application, totaling $99 for the first ten programs, $16 each for every additional application from 11–20, $20 each for every additional application from 21–30, and $26 each for every additional application after 30. The money adds up quickly.

About a month after applications are due, residency programs begin to invite students for interviews. In most specialties, interview invites (IIs) come randomly, on any day, at any hour. Upon receipt of an II, students enter the program's interview portal and select among the dates offered (usually two to five choices), taking into consideration interviews already scheduled at other programs and the time it takes to travel and attend the pre-interview social the night before. Unfortunately, every other student who is lucky enough to receive this II is also doing the same thing, and by nature of interviewer availability (each interviewer can only interview one interviewee), there are a limited number of slots open for each session.

For an applicant to schedule their preferred date, upon receipt of an II, they end up scrambling to log into the system to confirm attendance before another student can log in and snag the slot. For this reason, every notification that one gets on their phone during this II period can be extremely stress inducing, as it could indicate the need to consult their schedule and rapidly book a new interview, flights, hotels, etc. Since students often rotate through clerkships during this time and might be in the operating room, in the shower, or asleep when these invites come through, family members and significant others are often recruited to help monitor the email address. To make matters worse, some programs choose to offer more IIs than they have total interview slots, and the program fills within minutes on a first-come-first-serve basis, such that one might be boxed out of their dream program even before the interview date simply because they could not log into the system fast enough.

After all this, finally, when a student is fortunate enough to collect interviews and schedule slots fitting into their agenda, the interview season commences. Applying into orthopedic surgery, I knew attempting to break into one of the more competitive specialties would be a challenge, but from what my advisors had told me leading up to the opening of ERAS, I felt confident that I would be a formidable candidate. I had strong board scores and a few research awards under my belt to go along with a handful of publications in well-respected academic journals. I had a fair amount of medical school leadership experience and was elected social chair for the medical school during my senior year (an honor I held dearly for my ability to plan fun events like chicken nugget- and lime-themed parties). I heeded everyone's advice and applied to fifty-five programs in all (total cost: $1189), on the low end for others applying into this specialty.

By the end of the interview distribution period, however, I had been offered just seven interviews. Based on prior years' data, the "golden number of contiguous ranks" with which to feel comfortable matching into orthopedic surgery (i.e., 95% chance) was twelve. Because I had definitely not achieved this benchmark, I asked my department to make calls on my behalf to help secure a few more interviews. This was not an unreasonable appeal, and many departments did this preemptively to target programs of particular interest to students. While my home department had informed me that they would not be making these calls prior to the interview invitation period, now that I was in danger of not matching, I was told the calls would go out. Unfortunately for me, it was too little too late and nobody bit; the interviews had already been distributed. So, with time ticking until the first interviews were conducted, I attempted to take fate into my own hands. The results were variable.

I reached out to one program director (the individual in

charge of a residency program and the head of the selection committee) with whom I had worked previously, who gave me the canned response that "in any other year, they would have given me an interview." I emailed a physician, whom I had met years ago while in undergrad, who was able to talk to the selection committee on my behalf to secure an additional interview. The institution where my mentor previously worked also contacted me after their first round of interviews had been distributed to bring my total to nine. I had done what I could do, but still, I could not rest easy.

In the months leading up to the application, I had put a lot of thought into what I had hoped to get out of residency. I considered the quality of the training, resident camaraderie, and the research infrastructure. If I had been on this journey four years ago, I would have targeted programs ranked in the top ten of Doximity's Residency Navigator—the Hospital for Special Surgery, Harvard, and Rush—places with a brand to feed my ego regardless of where it took me. I know I would've done that because I did it for medical school, and four years before that, I did it for undergrad.

Lately, instead, I'd found myself thinking more about how wonderful of a time I had back in Georgia, living with Sarah and my parents during our COVID remote learning and being close to this support network, thinking over questions I had never pondered:

What does prestige even mean?

Who am I doing this for?

What is it that I'll want when I am finishing residency training?

It's hard to balance the priorities you have in the present day with those you anticipate you'll have five years in the future, where a wife and kids might be in the picture. I could imagine a scenario where a growing family was my reality, and if that were the case, would any of this really matter to me? The answer I had settled on was a resounding "no," and at this point in the process, I had hoped to land a position which would bring me closer to home, where Sarah—who would be going through this process the next year—would also be able to join me. In my mind, these opportunities were in the Raleigh area, Atlanta, and Nashville. Plus, and if all else failed, I could remain in Chicago.

After the interviews were distributed, and I only had one in the South, the most appealing cities to me had already been crossed off the list. I would be lying if I said there wasn't a mourning period for this future I had constructed in my mind, but in the aftermath of this bombshell, with only nine interviews total, I had bigger fish to fry. I recalibrated and convinced myself that I would be happy to match anywhere, to be an orthopedic surgeon waking up every day doing the job I had always dreamed of doing. That would be an accomplishment in itself, and certainly, that was not a given in my present situation. In any case, Chicago was still on the list, and I got excited about potentially establishing roots there and not having to do a long-distance relationship for a year or more. I looked at apartments on Zillow in my free time; I found some cheap furniture that we could refurbish for our first place; we looked into adopting an orange cat together.

When my interviews started, I learned that the structure of each day was not all that new to me. The interviews themselves differed marginally by specialty, and though I cannot speak in detail to anything other than the field of orthopedic surgery, these interviews were structured in one of two ways.

The traditional interview day was organized around three

thirty-minute interviews. During these, one could expect to be asked various behavioral questions covering generic topics:

"Tell me about yourself."

"Why do you want to go into orthopedics?"

"Tell me about a time you failed. What did you learn from this?

"What's an ethical dilemma that you have faced?"

"Describe a time when your opinion differed from others you have worked with. How did you remedy this?"

"What is your proudest achievement?"

The alternate interview structure included six or more eight-to-twelve-minute interviews, each typically centered around a theme—research, ethics, or orthopedic knowledge, for example. In any other non-COVID year, I would have attended these interviews by flying across the country to various programs, finding housing, and securing meals—all on my own dime. The cost of all this travel usually ran upwards of $10,000. Perhaps the one benefit of investing this money here was being able to see the programs up close and personal, touring the facilities, meeting faculty in person, and drinking free beer with the residents afterward. From what I'd heard, these experiences offered decent insight into the culture of the program, what they valued and what they didn't, and how well each cohort got along with one another. All of this was pertinent information in deciding where to spend the next three to seven years of one's life (five years for orthopedic surgery).

In the middle of the pandemic, though, since all in-person interviews had been canceled, every program around the country agreed to conduct interviews via virtual platforms. Most had subbed out the pre-interview social the night before with a Zoom happy hour where students were placed into breakout rooms with four other applicants and moved at fifteen-minute intervals into five consecutive resident rooms, slowly sipping on lagers off frame and asking and answering the same questions on a loop.

"Why don't we do introductions? Tell me your name, where you're from, where you went to school, and maybe a fun fact about yourself."

"Hi, my name is Sean. I'm originally from Suwanee, Georgia. I went to undergrad at Vanderbilt University. I'm at the University of Chicago right now. A fun fact about me is that I'm neighbors with Barack Obama."

By the third round I could recite all my colleagues' fun facts.

These sessions were always followed by the virtual interview in the morning. In preparation for these, I had spent over an hour carefully curating my room, throwing dirty clothes in places my front-facing camera could not see, taking down and replacing paintings, moving houseplants and candles, and buying a ring light. The goal was to look put together without trying too hard to look put together. I ended up with a background that was aesthetically pleasing to my male gaze, and from this higher ground, silently judged the choices of others: medical textbooks stacked on a bookshelf; unfinished woodworking projects transparently serving as a conversation starter; a skeleton looming in the corner which, in the best-case scenario, cost $50 on Amazon; even a black bedsheet pinned to the wall making the interviewee look like he was tuning in from the set of a snuff film.

My roommates and I had shared a Google Calendar of our interview dates with one another so as to avoid friendly fire of multiple people talking over each other's rehearsed answers through thin walls. To ensure a stable internet connection, we'd bought three 100-foot Ethernet cables, which zigzagged across the living room for months on end. Compared to the medical school application process, when the residency interview season ended, I had far fewer stories from the trail and a far worse understanding of the culture of each institution. From the tiny boxes on my computer screen, every program looked and felt the same. At the conclusion of the season, I was left with two months to tinker with my rank list prior to the official due date in early March. Given my specific situation and priorities, of the choices presented to me, I had a clear-cut number one. After this, most of the other programs either had red flags (malignant culture, lack of diversity, changes in leadership) or, more commonly, were located in places where they were the only major hospital system in the region and, as a result, would be difficult places for my partner to also match the following year: Palo Alto, Seattle, Ann Arbor, Milwaukee.

In this period following interviews, and to not invalidate the stable marriage match algorithm, programs are barred from initiating further post-interview communication (PIC) with students. If history has taught us anything, though, it is that programs cannot be trusted to play fair, and inevitably every year, many reach out to their favorite students via phone (so there is no paper trail) using vague language to convey their intended meaning:

"We are impressed by the quality of your application."

"You are a top candidate."

Some are even more to the point: "You are ranked to match."

More than a handful of students every year are the beneficiaries of this borderline unethical PIC, and of course, everybody applying wants this assurance going into Match Day. Hell, I wanted this information. It would have alleviated a ton of stress, though certainly not all of it because I was also aware that, every year, tragedies happened where programs reached out to applicants either directly via phone or indirectly through their mentors, letting them know they would be ranked highly, only for the applicant to ultimately fall past them on the rank list, or worse, not match at all. Both outcomes can only happen in the case of insincerity on the part of the hospital. This is where the decision tree involutes. Do I want PIC or not? If I do, is it genuine? If it's genuine, how does it factor into my rank list?

As it played out, I was not one of these lucky students anyway, and for all this criticism about program misconduct, students, for their part, also attempt to manipulate the narrative in their favor. Before rank lists are due, most craft letters to their top choice letting them know they are ranking them first. Because I had an obvious number one, I sent a letter to Northwestern hoping it might have some influence on where they might rank me. It's unclear how much any of this swayed anybody, but the psychology of this decision was on the side of the initiator. Everybody wants to feel wanted—it is a fundamental human quality—and program directors surely hoped to match students who were excited to be working for them, just as students surely wanted to attend programs that were willing to put on this display of affection.

Mind games aside, on the day that rank lists are officially due, every applicant and every program submit their respective lists to the governing body called the National Ranking Match Program (NRMP). I can only assume that, within nanoseconds of closing, the algorithm has already placed everybody into their stable marriages, but for reasons that I do not know, there is a two-week delay from when we click submit until the next contact from the NRMP. The communication that we do finally receive is at 11:00 a.m. on the Monday of the third week in March every year, a week which has been imaginatively named Match Week. In this email, we receive information telling us whether or not we matched. The verdict is a binary of yes or no without mention of where.

Those who receive a "yes" are guaranteed an employer next year in their chosen specialty, at a hospital to be revealed later that week. For those who are not so fortunate, there is an entirely separate system called the Supplemental Offer and Acceptance Program (SOAP), which attempts to place unmatched applicants across the nation into any unmatched residency spots. Sometimes, these positions are in the intended field of study, but more often than not, they are in other specialties and locations that are less desired (hence why the positions went unfilled in the first place). This process takes place over the few days following the Monday of Match Week, and after several rounds of new applications, interviews, and offers, many are still left without a job, including, in years past, multiple of my colleagues and friends. These students must make the difficult choice between taking a gap year to strengthen their resumes for application into the same specialty the following cycle, switching specialties, or dropping out of medicine and changing career paths entirely.

I had spent four years of my life waiting for this moment, and in all of the pageantry of Match Week, it was easy to forget just how ridiculous it was that a computer was the gatekeeper determining my fate, telling me whether or not I could be an orthopedic surgeon, even after all of these years of studying and sacrifice.

In the midst of this anger, fear, and anticipation, an email populated my phone telling me that I had matched. I breathed a huge sigh of relief. With only nine interviews, there was certainly an alternate dimension where the SOAP could have been my reality. Later that day, I looked at the national data published every year:

- 28% of all applicants applying pediatrics did not match pediatrics (11% for graduates from United States medical schools [US MD])
- 40% of all applicants applying family medicine did not match family medicine (13% US MD)
- 37% of all applicants applying internal medicine did not match internal medicine (15% US MD)
- 24% of all applicants applying emergency medicine (EM) did not match EM (15% US MD)
- 35% of all applicants applying psychiatry did not match psychiatry (15% US MD)
- 28% of all applicants applying OB/GYN did not match OB/GYN (16% US MD)
- 33% of all applicants applying orthopedics did not match orthopedics (25% US MD)
- 42% of all applicants applying neurosurgery did not match neurosurgery (26% US MD)
- 46% of all applicants applying general surgery did not match general surgery (27% US MD)
- 46% of all applicants applying anesthesia did not match anesthesia (30% US MD)
- 43% of all applicants applying plastic surgery did not match plastic surgery (30% US MD)
- 37% of all applicants applying otolaryngology did not match otolaryngology (32% US MD)

These figures were representations of real people who had decided that they wanted to dedicate their lives to the cause of others. They'd worked hard to excel in academics, passing qualifying exams and gaining acceptance into medical school. In lieu of a job, they'd decided to invest in this dream, taking on four more years of schooling and hundreds of thousands of dollars in student loans, unaware, like me, when entering that, every year, thousands of graduating MDs went unmatched. They entered medicine under the correct belief that the United States was in the midst of a physician shortage, but instead of the promise of a field that would welcome them with open arms, they were informed via email that the computer algorithm was unable to find them a stable marriage. Instead, they experienced the manifestation of the number of residency spots increasing just 1 percent annually despite medical school spots increasing more than 52 percent since 2002.

In spite of these bleak statistics, I had cleared this hurdle and could relax for a few more days. I put the fear behind me because the worst-case scenario had changed drastically. The nightmare had been avoided but still so much was to be revealed. The next communication from the NRMP came four days later. For additional reasons that I do not know, this happens at noon Eastern Time every year, not a second before, on the Friday known as Match Day.

On Match Day, every single medical school across the country hosts a blowout ceremony where students, families, and friends are invited. At some schools, when noon arrives, everybody hurriedly tears open their letters at the same time to collectively discover their fate. For others, each student must go up on a stage when their name is called to open the letter and read where they are contractually obligated to go, to have their reaction witnessed by all and live streamed to an online audience. At my school, we were allowed, mercifully, to silo off into small groups with our nuclear families and friends to celebrate or lament as needed.

The day itself was filled with butterflies. Again, because of COVID, our Match Day had been transitioned from the auditorium of Mitchell Hospital to an online platform. I had gathered with my closest friends in their home earlier that morning for brunch, attempting to settle my nerves with a Bloody Mary and a few strips of bacon. We signed into the Zoom link at 11:00 a.m. The following hour was filled with a slideshow of pictures: classmates goofing off, studying, sleeping in class. There were pictures of the group from nights on the town, field day, the boat cruise, working in the hospital; in each, we slowly watched ourselves age before our eyes. Four years older, four years wiser. We shared senior superlatives we had submitted to poke fun at every person in our class, but under this charade was a gnawing sensation that we just wanted to know where we were going. It had been a long four years filled with peaks and troughs, and our futures were being suspended before us somewhere in the cybersphere. As the minutes creeped nearer, we all watched the clock, sweating, anxious as the second hand twitched reluctantly.

I received a notification on my phone at noon and, with shaking hands, unlocked the screen. The email loaded and my eyes darted around searching for any words that might look familiar. What I saw surprised me. I didn't get my first choice. I didn't get my second choice. I didn't even get my third choice. I FaceTimed my parents and, in a stupor, told them where I had landed.

I had matched at the University of Washington in Seattle.

This was, for full disclosure, my sixth choice. When I learned this, I was in shock because the future I had built up in my mind had again been shattered in an instant. This was a program and city not just where I was going to start my career, but it was how I was going to experience the next twelve months and possibly the next five years of my life. The stress of what Sarah and I would have to do next year to get her to match there was already palpable, and when I called my mentor, he could hear it in my voice. I was not okay. When I hung up, I took a moment to collect my thoughts, immediately trying to rationalize this terrible irony that, at the end of the day, I had matched at the best program at which I had interviewed. It was a program that, years ago, I had identified as one of my favorites, located in a city where I had wanted to live. In an unexpected way, my hopes were met on Match Day in that the program was equally a revelation of my future and a reflection of my past. But it wasn't what I wanted; it didn't fit into my plan.

In the context of the match statistics, I felt conflicted in feeling any disappointment at being selected at all, let alone by this institution. I had, in fact, really enjoyed my interview day. I liked the depth and breadth of the training offered, what I knew of the resident culture, the program's commitment to diversity. For all of this, I felt grateful, but I also felt justified in my worry because the most important criteria of my "stable marriage" had not been fulfilled. It didn't seem fair that a computer algorithm would be expected to know this, and of course, I couldn't be surprised when it failed to take it into account.

Growing up, I was taught that everything happened for a reason. This was something that I internalized in real time, and when I finally arrived at the rebellious age where I felt more mature, debatably wiser, I started to form ideas of my own. I began to grapple with this concept, considering that faith alone may no longer be enough. I wanted and needed more. Why was there so much suffering in the world? What happened to good people when they died? Why was religion consistently corrupted into observable evil? Why did I have fucking Crohn's disease?

I spent a lot of time and energy trying to find the answers, and honestly, I don't think I ever did. For all of the bad in the world for which I never found reasons, I still believe that, in the face of human tragedy, all of this is not for nothing and that there is a plan outside the scope of my understanding which serves to make us all stronger individuals and more sympathetic, better humans. I am, after all, a person who believes that things happen for a reason—or, at least, I am a person who needs to believe that things happen for a reason. Perhaps this is because, on a much more insular scale, despite my doubts, in my life, when things had not followed the blueprint I had drafted, it had been easy for me to observe the blessings with which I was afforded in their place.

When I was applying to college, I knew where I wanted to go. My sister was two grades ahead of me, and when she was a junior in high school starting to look toward university, I tagged along and had my first taste of higher education. During my freshman year, far before my peers concerned themselves with these matters, I had found my dream school. Most days, I finished homework and prepared for tests, working toward this goal. This was what motivated me. I buried myself in books, and with each passing semester, I was getting closer. As the story goes, I didn't get into my first-choice college, and at the time, this ate away at me. There was a period where I was heartbroken, but after my time at Vanderbilt University, I knew that was where I was meant to be. It gave me friendships that will last for life. It challenged my understanding of race and privilege. It gained me acceptance into medical school, where I could pursue my passion of becoming a doctor.

Even still, my dream school was out there, and applying to medical school gave me another chance. This time, I scored an interview, but after many months on the waitlist, I never came off. Instead, I went to the University of Chicago, where I found a collection of incredible mentors and friends, and most importantly, somebody with whom to do life. For all the circumstance, every decision, each success and failure that had led me to this place, I knew that this was where I was meant to be.

The story this time felt so familiar. I had created worlds and had them erased without my approval. Even still, I was hopeful, like before, that this was all for a reason, that this was where I was meant to go, but it scared me that I did not yet know for sure. In the context of everything else happening outside the narrow world of medicine, though, it seemed silly that this even mattered. There were days when I wanted to tell myself to stop being so selfish and just be thankful. Be thankful that my parents were healthy, that I had a roof over my head, that there was a medication out there allowing me to take a shit in the morning without discomfort. Be thankful for all the moments of perfection in my life, that there were things as beautiful as the complexity of a pinecone sitting on the ground beside a park bench, or a temperate breeze in my face coming off a lake that looked like an ocean, or somebody playing the trombone in a parking garage on a Sunday afternoon in April. And I knew I was getting there, day by day.

18

SOMEWHERE IN BETWEEN

So while thousands of Jack's Todays will, to an outsider from far away, begin to look like a complete picture, Jack spends each moment of his actual reality in one unremarkable Today pixel or another. Jack's error is brushing off his mundane Wednesday and focusing entirely on the big picture, when in fact the mundane Wednesday is the experience of his actual life.

—Tim Urban, "Life is a Picture, But You Live in a Pixel," *Wait But Why*

I GRADUATED MEDICAL SCHOOL ONLINE. The dean recorded an introduction over webinar. We had hired the US Surgeon General to give the commencement address. When my picture flashed across the screen, my family texted me balloon emojis.

My graduations before this were so full of clichés. I would sit in an auditorium crammed next to hundreds of others wearing sweaty polyester gowns. When summoned, we would scamper onto the stage and awkwardly shake hands with five people whom we had never met. If we were fortunate, our last names wouldn't be butchered in the process and nobody would take grainy photos of us on their iPads afterward. It's funny how my perspective on graduating has changed. In elementary school, I got to pretend to be a grown-up for a day. In high school, I felt like I had already grown up. College was a bittersweet affair.

Four years ago, I would have never guessed that this is how it would have ended. I had spent the past month at home while my friends traveled the world. We had all flown back to Chicago that weekend to pack our belongings into cardboard boxes and say goodbye one last time. On the day of the ceremony, we drove out to the suburbs to celebrate as a small group. A friend had connected her laptop to the TV with an HDMI cable so we could tune in at 11:00 a.m. sharp, and all of us brought different side dishes to eat. This event didn't have any of the clichés that characterized prior graduations, but as anticlimactic as it was, it somehow felt more significant. No virus could take away the fact that we had accomplished something incredible, and even though our names were called out over the speakers of a computer, I could not help but feel proud. In spite of the imposter syndrome, burnout, and long nights spent studying, I had come out the other side and lived to tell the tale. I knew that this day was the culmination of hundreds if not thousands of average days. Days spent buried in books, under a microscope, stressing out over product yields in organic chemistry lab, red-eyed over a mound of piling secondary applications. It was earned through flashcards and Q-banks, standardized patient encounters and sub-internships. I didn't get to walk across a stage or throw my cap in the air, but I didn't need it to feel that same sense of wonder as I did when I backpacked my way through Europe or stood atop the Great Wall, the wind thrashing my face as I stared out at Mongolia and China for what felt like an eternity.

From a bird's-eye view, it is easy to appreciate the big days for what they are: moments of anticipation, happiness, the culmination of months to years of hype. These moments are exponentially heightened when they manage to meet our wildest expectations: the day of our marriage or the birth of our kids or even when we get that white coat we've been dreaming about since we were little. It's natural to get swept up in these achievements, and I choose to celebrate these days for their rarity because seldom are triumphs tied together with such neat ends. One day, though, we all must hop on a plane home from Europe or climb down the Great Wall. The honeymoon eventually comes to an end, and while the nature of the emotions experienced on the big days can be a pinnacle of intoxicating happiness, they are, by the nature of emotions, fleeting. I feel happy because I know sadness, or at least the absence of happiness. I must return to a baseline not by choice but by default.

Life is a series of in-betweens bookended by major events: graduations, promotions, births, and weddings. For most of my training, I have looked toward the future with a steadfast intensity because it has always seemed so promising. In doing so, I dedicated myself to the sacrifice of todays in search of a better tomorrow. As a premed, I just wanted to be in medical school. During the preclinical years, I just wanted to be on the wards. As a clinical student, I thought if I could just be a resident, then life would be that much better. It seems like every resident wants to be a junior attending, and every junior attending wants to be a senior attending, too. It doesn't stop, but the crazy thing is that I don't think life gets any easier with these graduations, it just gets different along the way. In the time spent waiting for the next best thing, I'm sure I've missed a lot about what was right in front of me.

Maybe the only reason quarantine had an upside, and something I feel infinitely grateful for, was the amount of time spent in the present. The world had stopped spinning for nearly a year, and as it slowed, so did I. I went home with Sarah and spent afternoons on the golf course watching my dad fist pump the air with the drop of every long putt. I built bonfires and roasted s'mores while my mom shared stories that I was finally old enough to hear. I got to see my sister become a dog mom, and I reconnected with my oldest friends, looking on in awe over late-night conversations in a hot tub as these people whom I'd known only as kids grew into fully realized humans before me.

As the end of my time in Georgia drew nearer, life began to feel more real. I started worrying again about sub-internships and away rotations and finally starting residency and what that meant, but in returning to the world of school and jobs and Sunday scaries, I tried to take with me a mindfulness for the present: saying grace before dinner, sharing stories from patient care with my roommates each night, writing a line in a journal before slipping off to sleep. While I was sacrificing moments of potential energy to be on this journey, I started to better appreciate the experience of existing in the now.

On my last night in Chicago, for the first time since I can remember, I didn't want a big moment. I went to the grocery store, bought some pizzas, and invited over my best friends. I put an NBA playoff game on the TV that I didn't care about and sat there on a broken couch in their company for hours. I didn't want to talk about anything significant or the changes that were on the horizon. I just wanted to be surrounded by my favorite people in a place that I will always think back to with reverence, shooting the shit about who knows what, feeling comfortable and happy and at home.

I don't really understand how time seems to move at two speeds. Some days it flies by, and other days it drags, but in both, there never is a choice in how fast it moves. On the wards, there were days that I wish I could have fast-forwarded through to the evening, and as the end of my time in medical school hurtled to a finish, I wanted so desperately to slow things down, bargaining with the gods for one more of everything. One more class party. One more Social Rounds. One more senior skit. I wouldn't have even been greedy; I just wanted one last night on the third floor of a walk-up apartment on Ellis Avenue where doing nothing was always doing something.

The next morning, though, I waved bye to John, asleep on the sofa, and boarded an early morning flight out of Midway International. Tess, Rob, and Kelly went north to their new apartments in the city. Emily headed east toward Philly; Maya K and Henry were southbound to Atlanta; and Bobby and Maya R drove a U-Haul west in the direction of Denver.

For all the uncertainty and confusion, transitions don't have to be bad. I look up and see a lot of good happening around me. I recently got engaged to the love of my life. I'm starting my first real job in a couple weeks. Two of my closest friends bought a home together. For all the change, so much beauty has come out of it. I found an amazing support network that is worth missing, I stole time from the world and spent it with my family in Georgia, and I learned how to be a doctor in the process.

The possibility the imminent future presents is both exciting and overwhelming. What comes next is a new kind of potential, and though I have no idea what to make of the depths I am entering, I am ready. Scared, yes. Hesitant, of course. But mostly, I am ready.

ACKNOWLEDGMENTS

Nothing in my life has been accomplished in a vacuum, and this book is no different. First, thank you to my wife, Sarah. She has been a sounding board for countless passages in this book and a caring partner through the *experiences* of those passages. I remember early on, when we had only been dating for a few months, shortly after I was diagnosed with Crohn's disease and started taking Humira, I had to go to the main campus to have blood drawn, the results of which would essentially tell me if I was responding appropriately to the medication. I told Sarah I was headed to campus to have several tests run, and she canceled all of her afternoon appointments and insisted on being there, sitting with me in the waiting room, and walking me back home. I feel so lucky to be the recipient of her affection.

Thank you to my parents and older sister, Georgia, for providing more support than I could have ever dreamed was possible and for encouraging me to write in the days before this book was even an idea, when my content was barely readable and certainly not entertaining. Medical school and residency have taken me thousands of miles from home and caused me to miss more family reunions, holidays, and vacations than I would like to admit, but I have never felt too far away with them on the other end of the phone.

This book in its current form also would not have been

possible without contributions from my incredibly kind and talented editors, Martha Calderaro and Kasia Kalinowska, and I am endlessly appreciative of their insight.

I am somewhat regretful that research could not have been emphasized more in this book despite its being a large part of who I was as a medical student. Over four years, I spent hundreds of hours poring over chart reviews, editing code, writing scientific articles, and traveling to conferences. Perhaps more important, though, were the hours spent exchanging emails and meeting with my research mentor, Dr. Michael J. Lee.

The more I have progressed through residency, the more I have come to understand that every investment an attending physician makes in a medical student requires some sort of sacrifice on their part (e.g., being away from the operating room, clinic, or family). It is incredible to look back on medical school and see just how much Dr. Lee was willing to invest in me, my career, and my personal development. During MS4, Dr. Lee gave me perhaps the best pieces of advice I have ever received:

1. *If you're ever pimped about a statistic in the literature (e.g., What percentage of anterior cervical discectomy and fusions typically go on to nonunion? What is the rate of infection after a multilevel lumbar spine fusion?), answer with a numerical range instead of a single number (i.e., 2–7% risk of nonunion, 5–10% risk of infection). Doing so substantially increases the chance of being correct and makes wrong answers closer to being right answers.*
2. *"Pony up" and propose to Sarah.*

He has been a man after whom I hope to model my career and personal life.

Finally, many thanks to all my past teachers, who helped fuel a curiosity that led me to medicine. To all my patients, who have made me a better doctor and human. And to you, the reader, for being a willing audience for my musings.

ABOUT THE AUTHOR

Doctor, writer, and coed flag football intramural champion Sean Pirkle has studied in the libraries of many US cities. He earned his bachelor's degree from Vanderbilt University before attending medical school at the University of Chicago. Afterward, he moved to Seattle to complete his orthopedic surgery residency at the University of Washington. An accomplished researcher, he has published numerous scientific articles on surgical techniques and outcomes, and his opinion editorials have been featured in the *Journal of Bone and Joint Surgery,* the premier journal in orthopedics. In his free time, he enjoys spending time with his wife and cats. *Somewhere in Between* is his first book.